ANY OTHER SONG

Executive Producer: *Richard A. Weimer*
Production Editor; Cover and Text Design: *Marlise Reidenbach*
Illustrator: *S. J. Nash*

Any Other Song

a plea for holistic communication

E. J. Daniel

Robert J. Brady Co.

A Prentice-Hall Publishing and
Communications Company

Bowie, Maryland 20715

Any Other Song: A Plea for Holistic Communication
Copyright © 1980 by Robert J. Brady Co. All rights reserved. No part of this publication may be reproduced or transmitted in any form or by any means, electronic or mechanical, including photocopying and recording, or by any information storage and retrieval system, without permission in writing from the publishers. For information, address Robert J. Brady Co., a Prentice-Hall Publishing and Communications Company, Bowie, Maryland 20715.

Library of Congress Cataloging in Publication Data

Daniel, E J
    Any Other Song.

    1.   Medical personnel and patient.   2.   Nurse and patient.   3.   Interpersonal communication.   4.   Communication in medicine.   5.   Holistic medicine.   I.   Title.
R727.3.D36   610.69'6   79-24892
ISBN 0-87619-460-9

Prentice-Hall International, Inc., London
Prentice-Hall of Australia, Pty., Ltd., Sydney
Prentice-Hall of India Private Limited, New Delhi
Prentice-Hall of Japan, Inc., Tokyo
Prentice-Hall of Southeast Asia Pte. Ltd., Singapore
Whitehall Books, Limited, Petone, New Zealand
Printed in the United States of America

80 81 82 83 84 85 86   10 9 8 7 6 5 4 3 2 1

*warm and endless loving thanks to
Judy, Beth and Karin*

CONTENTS

Foreword
Prelude

Toccata   *1*
Interlude   *127*
Fugue   *131*

Postlude

FOREWORD

In preparing for a career in any of the helping professions, the student is exposed to a wide variety of learning experiences, all geared to provide the body of knowledge and understanding considered essential for practice. Some of the most sensitive and difficult concepts for the student and practitioner are the dynamics of emotional distress—of anger, dependency, regression and manipulation. *Any Other Song* will provide the reader with a unique opportunity to experience the torture and frustration of clients in their pleas for help. The interweaving of objective clinical data documented by health professionals, and the client's descriptions of her experiences and feelings, are presented in a compelling manner.

    The book was written for students and practicing health professionals, but the nature of the dialogue provides a moving experience for all who read it.

Grace L. Davis, R.N., M.A.
Director of Nursing Education
Children's Hospital, San Francisco

Spring 1979

PRELUDE

Any Other Song is an extensive case study that delves into the relatively unexplored world of the patient-in-crisis and the all too common miscommunication between patient and health professional. It is hoped this text may prove an invaluable tool for the professional seeking to grow in understanding of the at-risk client. Not to discount or berate the variable effectiveness of medical intervention, my intent rather has been to point out the absolute necessity of seeing the patient as a *whole person,* who adapts, heals and functions as an individual. Becoming involved with the Person is an inherent trait of the helping profession, but the empathetic caring has never been a quality to demand.

My purpose is not to point the finger at any one individual, but to explore communication patterns and, through the discussion questions, to aim for a more edifying, holistic approach to the patient. Please realize that the occasionally strong language and diverse perceptions are those of the patient-in-crisis, and should be so interpreted. To protect those involved, names and some circumstances have been altered. The following are briefly explained, for clarification:

From the lab—secretaries Spence and Darley,
R. N.s Annie and Kelly;
Kathy's husband—Ted; his classmates and their mutual friends Lindy, Nance, Jo and Ron;

Any Other Song

Psych ward—R.N.s Jude, Patty, Braye, Cory, and Sable,
        MHAs Jack, Lou, and Greg;
ER R.N.s—Julie, Brenda, Karin, Jourdie, J.J., and Amy.

Most of us involved have gone on to other places. Since these events, many may have even forgotten—pretending to go on as though it all really didn't matter. Some of us, though, will remember forever.

For their support, I would like to thank: Grace Davis, R.N., M.A., for encouraging me to pursue publication; Elizabeth Richardson, R.N., M.Ed., for listening; and Juliene Lipson, R.N., Ph.D., for "being there."

E. J. Daniel
July 1979

TOCCATA

ONE

Mom first took me to the doctor about my headaches when I was in the fourth grade. I don't exactly remember complaining of them all the time then, or for that matter, at any time then. I just ended up sitting in the doctor's mustard yellow office one stifling afternoon hearing him ramble in a very condescending manner—assuring Mom that nothing was really wrong with me. I suppose she had gotten pretty worried to take me in to see him in the first place, as illness and physicians were not high priority. Since he couldn't find anything, Crew-Cut presumed the cause must be tension—"when things don't go your way"—implying I was prone to extreme emotions. At any rate, that answer obviously satisfied Mom, and for the rest of my life, whenever I had a headache, she would say, "Why, something must not be going your way, honey."

That's probably why I was so relieved—genuinely happy, in fact—that the headache I got this time was real. At least, the doctors thought so. I didn't know what the consequences would be, but I do so love adventures and life had been terribly boring. That wasn't exactly true, because I'd taken on a part-time counseling job in addition to the medical research clerking in a lab (white coat and all), and was very busy, though not with my life's career. My teaching credentials had landed me not the long-awaited school contract, but a tremendous position as a secretary: "Kathy, can't

Any Other Song

you type this correctly?" Klutz. "Would you go find the records on this patient—now!" Gopher. "You wouldn't understand the procedure anyway, so don't ask." Dumb shit. But jumping into the schools just to replenish my damaged ego was turning out to be a not-so-clever maneuver. I had no sooner settled into the chaotic elementary system, trying to develop my own program for the behavior-disordered slow readers, than I caught the "pediatric crud." Having battled the bug for three weeks, I was finally allowed a weekend reprieve before being hit with the most incredible headache—right in the middle of a Monday morning class. I lasted until midafternoon when my motherly supervising teacher let me stagger out and drive home in a mental fog, having almost overdosed on aspirin in an attempt to get rid of the pain. My reward for making it home intact was dry heaves that exacerbated my raging headache. It hurt so bad I cried, which only made it worse. When Ted dragged home from classes and found me crouched in a corner of the bed, lights out, he promptly packed me up and deposited me at the hospital emergency room. It was 8:00. Half an hour later we were finally escorted into the glossy, gray-tiled examining room where, a mere hour later, an intern decided to see what was wrong with Kathy. Nice of him to volunteer.

You know, you have an S4! *That's terrific. But Ted didn't bring me down here for a cardiology exam. It's my head that hurts, not my heart.*

Then, because he didn't know what was wrong, he sent me upstairs for a series of x-rays. Ted waited with me through the tedious chest, skull and sinus films (might as well have been total body films for the time involved). The radiology department was eerily deserted by that hour, each footstep echoing up and down the darkened, fixative-reeking corridors. Back down the elevator to the foggy cubicle. In the incessant din of the ER, I was acutely aware of Ted's subdued silence.

> Would that I was summers past, secure in the branches of my childhood willow, rocking gently in the warm, mellow breeze, any afternoon, pleasantly alone.

Hi there! *This must be the ENT resident.* He whisked in, looked in my eyes, pressed around on my forehead, Does this hurt? Does that hurt? *and departed. He looked terribly sleepy behind his glasses and crumpled mustache, which nicely matched his surgical greens. Before I had time to mull over anything else, the intern wandered back in.* Your films are normal. Why don't you just go home and sleep it off? Take some of these, and here are some suppositories. *Even in my stagnated mental state, I wasn't impressed with this visit to the ER. As he urged us out the door, I thought maybe the codeine would help, after all. It was 1 AM. Time flies when you're having fun.*

On Wednesday, Spence said that I looked like shit. Strange, but that was exactly how I felt, but I wasn't sure if it was due to all the codeine I'd been scarfing down that wasn't working, or because of the raging headache that had persisted into a nightmare. Everything had been getting cloudy, and my outside wasn't letting me be seen. The ENT-in-green on Monday had said that if I still had a headache, to come back and see him Tuesday. So I did, and he peered again inside my head to study a part of me. After looking at the same x-rays with the department chief, he told me again that they were normal films, even though there was an "opaque area" where my frontal sinus should be. I just wanted to get it over. He looked at me funny then, and said he thought I should get a neurology consult. By then it was too late to be seen in clinic, so I was supposed to report back to the Emergency Room. I mumbled "sure," fumbled out of clinic, but was too tired to sit for eons in the zoo again. So I went home.

And it came to pass that in the latter days, part of me would self-destruct. All those-in-white watched and noted, nodding agreement as outside she became another. But i was inside, and no one saw me.

Otolaryngology note: headache—persistent pain, temporal area and frontal area, since 10:30 AM yesterday, without relief from codeine. Sinus films normal. Question tension headache, not sinus headache. Refer to neurology for further evaluation.

So when things kept getting slower and my boggy appearance refused to go into remission, those-at-the-hospital sent me down to Walk-In Clinic to see the neurologist, or whatever. I had only been in the chair a few minutes before a comfortably dressed nurse in

Any Other Song

levis and clogs beckoned me back into an examining room. Good thing I was wearing my lab coat; it had my name on it and I didn't want to be confused with anyone.

Do you always talk this slow? *Hardly! Not me. I'm energetic and outgoing, a jock, a funny lady. Can't you tell?* Look at the wall. Raise your shoulders. Scrunch your eyebrows. Smile. Hey, c'mon and smile! *It was making me nervous having to be examined by her. She stared intently at me, in me, through me, with her big tinted glasses.* Grit your teeth. *After looking piercingly in me again she drifted away, leaving me vegetating on a chair she'd sat me on after her interview so that I wouldn't tilt off the examining table. I was still in my lab coat. Why I seemed to be more together at other times than I was then I couldn't figure out, but on that sterile Beta-dyne afternoon it didn't really matter.*

Just before I thought I might pass out, the Nurse Practitioner smiled back into the room bringing with her a wire-rimmed, white-jacketed doc. He was too small, and I was glad to be sitting, since short men make me feel especially gargantuan.

Hi. Look over at the spot on the wall for me, please. *I started to ask him why he was whispering, but I really didn't care. It was irritating when they kept asking me to smile, since that was the last thing I felt like doing. Things weren't funny; they were curious, especially when this jerk had to go through the same song and dance the NP had just done. He should have believed her. As they withdrew into the hallway, leaving the lights inside dimmed, I began wondering why I'd bothered to go down there anyway. Because earlier the ENT had scared me with his strange expression, and Spencer said I'd slowed down too much to work. Or something. The silence they left me in grew more strange.*

Kathy, they want to get another consult on you because your affect is a little weird. Since it's late, we have to have you seen in the ER. Can you walk over there alright? *Before I'd processed what she meant, she was escorting me out of Medical B floating down the hall toward Emergency. I wished desperately that I could have known her some other way than as a patient to a nurse. I mean, after all, I was a real person, and could be fun to be with—except for now. Only she wasn't reading me inside, I didn't think, to know that I appreciated all her concern and attention. I wasn't flat, really—just my emotions were. I tried to show her I was alright, sort of, but just couldn't.* Why don't you just sit over here, and I'll get things arranged with the nurses in back. Will you be alright? *I nodded, trying to tell her "thank you," but nothing came out. The motley conglomeration in the smoke-cured waiting room just stared. You'd have thought they'd never seen a lab coat before. Why don't you just keep glued to that TV and pretend I'm not even here. Excellent.*

Kathy? *Me, dummy. Get up and walk toward the smiling nurse. Walk carefully into the brightly lit hallway and don't bump the door or they'll really know you're not together. I thought I was really trying. Those-in-white, though, look at you differently when you're labeled for a neuro consult, gently guiding you wherever, talking ever so calmly, watching—silent and intent. Back into a curtained cubicle, rerun of Monday, dimmed and gray. So tired.*

Hi! I'm Dr. Bearl. Hear you have a headache. For how long? *Too long, too much, too painful. He looked like a doctor, balding because his brain needed all the energy, beer gut bulging in a wrinkled paisley shirt, with dingy white sta-crumpled pants. He proceeded to conduct another neuro exam with a few added tricks he pulled out of his little black bag. I kept trying to steady myself on the table edge, but when he left, I thought I might fade off into another time and place. It reminded me of the hours I'd spent in the campus infirmary for observation after my diving accident. The nurses had gotten me all settled in bed but, checking on me later, found me dressed, wrapped up in a blanket, sitting in the chair and staring out the window. Same distant feeling without reason.*

Bearl reentered with the short, bearded chief resident and some other doc wading in behind wearing her polyester lab coat and looking like she'd just stepped out of the fifties.

Look at the wall there for me, please. *The little spot on the gray wall I was supposed to be studying in the dark became less and less interesting, as each doc took turns looking inside my eyes, exchanging glances, nodding and mumbling agreement. They were making me feel like one of those racy kaleidoscopes, and I was curious to know why they were so engrossed with whatever it was they saw inside. Those-in-white kept looking from eye to eye not telling me what they saw, but it sure wasn't me. How could they know me? Those skull and chest x-rays couldn't find me. Nobody was talking to me. And those-in-white floated back out leaving me to my own reveries and empty explanations.*

> Consultation note: Kathy is a 23 y/o white female with a chief complaint of headache of 3 days' duration. On Monday, patient awoke with a bilateral frontal headache. She never had a headache like this in her life. This has persisted over the past 3 days. Aspirin and codeine do not alter her headaches. They are exacerbated by movement, lying down, coughing and sneezing. Patient reports to

Any Other Song

have "flulike" syndrome the past 2 weeks which was markedly improved prior to this headache onset. At that time, she had a "stuffy nose" and minimally elevated temp of 100. Associated with her headache, patient has a "spaced-out" feeling and dizziness, nausea with some dry heaves. Patient has had headaches in the past but attributed them to the pill, and they were always helped with ASA. Her general appearance indicates acute illness.

When a clerk from admissions came into my deserted room, I realized that those-in-white weren't going to let me go home. It made me feel trapped and frightened being admitted without even knowing why or for how long. At least before I sort of knew when I went to see the orthopedist that I was hospitalized for my wracked back. At that time I'd endured 24-hour traction for five days. Then those-in-white transferred me from the infirmary to the county hospital for a myelogram (that unbearable x-ray performed on a multi-tilt table so the dye injected into the spine can saturate the defective discs). Ted said I looked ghastly afterwards. I thought I'd died. A little glib about the surgery they scheduled me into the next day, I looked upon it as another adventure. When I finally came out of the anesthesia two days later, I figured there was more to it than I'd thought. Like, they were happy to have saved the nerves in my leg so I could walk. I was stunned. But because of that little episode I realized I was more important to Ted than I'd thought. He gave up the swim team just to see me every day while I was hospitalized. I wondered where he was this time . . .

Are you alright dear? Why don't you undress and I'll be back in a minute to take your vitals. *She watched me for awhile as I sat on the edge of the bed, then left me again to my zombied dullness. Apparently the staff had already been briefed, as this nurse seemed inappropriately nervous, curious and intense. I stared at the hospital gown, a murky green in the dimness of twilight. What in hell was I doing there? I come to work, go to follow-up clinic, and then I don't get to go home. There wasn't time to get oriented. Things weren't making sense. And where was Ted? But I was too pulpy and lethargic to do anything about it.*

Open your mouth, dear. Then we need to weigh you. *The floor was freezing as I stood up. I was afraid I might bite the thermometer in half. That'd be cute.* Are you alright? Now, I know this is going to be uncomfortable, but. . . . *If I was "just fine" I don't imagine I'd be here. The aide watched on as the RN shot a floodlight into my eyes and I braced against the head of the bed.* They are dilated. *As though she hadn't believed the docs.* Hey—why don't you get all *the other aides and nurses from the whole ward, and turn this into a carnival side show. Honestly! Being on a general medical floor maybe explained the staff's curiosity. I crawled into the icy chlorine sheets as the nurses scurried out of the mud-brown room. You can always tell when something's wrong. Things that used to be so sweet turn sour, and everything else seems dead. Everything that ever mattered, anyway.*

I felt sadly alone and God seemed very distant. It didn't matter either that Ted finally showed up, a paler shade of paste.

Kathy! What's going on? *Appropriate question, Ted.*

Did you call Jo?

No, but I will. What are they doing? *Strike two.*

Well, you're the medical student. You tell me! Have to catch ya later. Things are too slow . . .

As Ted sat at my bedside, in strolled what could have passed for neurology grand rounds, only it seemed a bit late. The Freudian band leader asked Ted to "leave us alone for awhile." The impending scrutiny by all those-in-white became frightening.

> Neurology: 23-year-old school teacher, medical student's wife, admitted with 3-day history of severe headache. Had flulike illness 2 weeks ago, with sore throat, fever, "stuffy head" which gradually resolved. This past weekend felt well enough to go out and went to work on Monday. About 10 AM patient had onset of severe bitemporal headache with dry heaves, vertigo. Seen in Emergency Room, referred to ENT, sinus films normal. Headache has persisted and is described as sharp bitemporal pain markedly worsened by moving head, sneezing, coughing or lying down. Has not eaten for 3 days. Marked change in personality since Monday with listlessness, dullness, apathy, irritability, and slow movements. No recently documented chills or fever. Denies blurred vision, decreased strength on one side, decreased sensation. Feels generally weak and unsteady on her feet. By history from husband, has occasional tension headaches, but never anything like this. No previous history for seizures or migraine. Was exposed to youngster who died from encephalitis in early winter. Disc margins are blurred but can appreciate venous pulsations. Sways while walking but is able to tandem. My impression is an organic headache. Consider subarachnoid hemorrhage secondary to an aneurysm, encephalitis, tumor (including intraventricular with obstruction), venous obstruction, abscess.

I was amazed at how far removed I seemed from everything when Jo and Lindy whispered into the dimness, their eyes wide. Inside I craved their attention and concern, but outside thought they were

Any Other Song

being very melodramatic. After all, I only had a headache, and was a little dull. No big deal. But they behaved as though something else was wrong; I just hoped Jo could differentiate well, and really see me inside. We'd known each other so long—she'd instructed me, admonished me, listened to me, cried with me—longer than Ted. And she knew me in a way he never could. He was always so busy lately, so preoccupied; I'd been attempting to reconstruct my life with less of him involved—not by choice, but out of necessity. You can only solo so long. I deduced God was teaching me to be the one who needed somebody for a change. In high school, I'd always been "the rock" because everyone could dump on me when their worlds fell apart. They always said how neat it was to have someone like me for a friend. The only problem was, there didn't seem to be anyone for me to run to, though I suppose I never could have let go anyway. I felt it would have ruined my reputation for being strong. Jo was about the only person who'd bothered to know me; she could see when something was wrong, even when I said nothing was. For all the time she'd spent on me, I had tried to return even a shadow of that understanding when she had needed it, trying to keep part of her intact when she lost the one person who'd meant so much to her. Sometimes, though, it's really hard to show how much you care. You just sort of believe the love's there. She and Lindy sat on opposite sides of my bed where I lay mummified on starched sheets.

It's weird how everyone keeps looking in my eyes.

Wish I had my instruments with me so I could see what the docs are all excited about. *I guess I made them nervous, and as they prayed over me, I was someplace else.*

Jo squeezed my blanketed leg, expressing what she couldn't put into words, and then they left me. In the ensuing silence I nearly cried, but my outside wouldn't let me. I was too lost in the dimness by then.

> Attending note: 23-year-old woman with 2 to 3 weeks viral URI symptoms and now 3-day throbbing headache with retching. Husband describes clearcut change in personality, difficulty sleeping, dull and unsteady gait. Also, she describes headache much worse when lying down. Only prior neurological problems—laminectomy and injured neck 2 years ago in diving accident, with residual headaches. No significant fever or chills. Child at school where she works had measles encephalitis and died 6 wks ago. Physical exam revealed a dull, slow, irritable woman with pain and photophobia; BP 110/70. Gait mildly ataxic, can tandem but can't hop, pupil movement normal, but I think she has papilledema bilaterally.

E. J. Daniel

Arms normal, but diffuse weakness (question poor effort) of legs. Doubt meningitis, but signs and symptoms indicate increased pressure and I suspect hydrocephalus. Need immediate neurosurgical consult and decide concerning angiogram.

TWO

Hey. How are you feeling? A different nurse had strolled in to watch things get dizzier and less real, wheeling in the blood pressure stick with her. She left the cuff on my arm. *Sorry, but we have to check on you every hour. Later this evening a couple more doctors will be coming by to examine you. Are you alright?* She really was concerned, but I wasn't thrilled about more flashlights and more docs introducing themselves just to be forgotten in my fadedness. I felt very isolated, and was beginning to get a little scared.

It must have been a couple of hours after Ted had gone when a sandy-red-haired jock sauntered in, grinning like a cheshire cat, and wearing a bleached neon lab coat.

Hello, young lady. I'm Dr. Darius. Some headache you've got, huh? He was actually fun to visit with. At least he seemed interested in me, joking about spouses and medical school as he looked inside, too. Before I realized it, the jock had melted away, leaving me alone again.

> Neurosurgery consult: Kathy is a 23 y/o white female with 2½ days headache of sudden onset at 10 AM Monday, followed by dry heaves, nausea and dizziness, all of which have persisted. Associated personality change of listlessness and apathy. Headache is bifrontal, bitemporal. Patient is afebrile, but does complain of

Any Other Song

> photophobia since that time. Sinus films were wnl on Monday. Had flu one week ago. She is alert, oriented and cooperative with normal speech except for apathy. No venous pulses seen—query early disc margin blurring. Well-healed laminectomy midline incision with chronic low back pain. R/o subarachnoid hemorrhage, posterior fossa midline tumor with hydrocephalus and encephalitis. Suggest brain scan in AM and then evaluate for next step.

After the battery of quiz sessions, I began wondering if I was even keeping my story coherent. I was so tired, and the questions those-in-white asked were too picky; I almost said "yes" to anything just to get rid of them. If they would only talk to that first intern I'd seen on Monday before I got too confused. I couldn't remember if I was telling them everything I should or if I was forgetting some things, and it was too hard to try and convince them that what they were seeing wasn't me. Maybe if they asked that NP in clinic . . .

The room had been turning more blue-black as night etched on, the only light a dim shaft from the hall piercing into the curtained darkness. I wondered, in a distant sort of way, what God had in mind for me this time; He was being so elusive. How was I supposed to make any sense out of anything?

Excuse me. I apologize for the late hour, but Dr. Forster felt it was imperative for me to see you tonight. *Ichabod Crane himself stood over my numb body, continuing to mumble. It was appropriate enough for midnight.*

> Nuclear Medicine: R-handed female, wife of second-year medical student. Six weeks ago exposed to encephalitis. No sequellae. Two to 3 weeks ago had URI with cough, nasal congestion. Several days ago had onset of gradually progressive headache—did not begin as sudden or instantaneous. Associated nausea, irritability. Do not think veins of fundi are engorged and pulsations are present. However, disc margins are slightly blurred. My impression is venous sinus obstruction, with some secondary mild bleeding, due to birth control pills. Cannot rule out meningitis, abscess, but doubt subarachnoid hemorrhage or tumor.

Inside, I was so drowsy, but I quickly discovered that it was easier not to fall asleep as my nerves couldn't take the jolts from being awakened every hour getting my blood pressure taken and my eyes checked.

> Nursing notes: 1:30 AM. Patient's arms and legs weak, pupils dilated but equal; she is reactive and oriented.

3:30 AM. Arms weaker than legs, pupils unchanged, speech sluggish, headache back, slight nuchal rigidity. Resident notified.
5:15 AM. Nailbeds cyanotic, color dusky; cold, clammy. Oxygen administered. Resident called.

I must have drifted off to sleep since I was jolted awake with that terrifying sensation of falling off a cliff. The nurse had just popped in on her rounds, looked at me, and scurried back into the too-bright hallway, calling for the respiratory team. Then I noticed my outside, all cramped and hyperventilating. I couldn't understand how I'd gotten so out-of-breath, and being unable to get enough air made me even more panicky.

Has this ever happened to you before? *Oh, sure! I do it all the time for sheer excitement—I just look scared. Those-in-white plugged me into the hissing oxygen and began massaging my grotesquely cramped arms and ice-blue feet. Dr. Bearl finally arrived, half awake, blurry-eyed.*

She's just a little apprehensive. She'll be alright. You really didn't need to wake me up. *I angrily studied the grungy ceiling, but the bonneted respiratory nurse really knew that I was terrified about everything. She kept checking on me, coaxing me to slow down my breathing, working out the cramps in my arms and hands. I groaned in pain.*

Oh! I'm sorry. That still hurts, huh? You're doing just fine! *The oxygen continued to whistle in my face through the clear green tubes plugged into my nostrils.* Can you open your eyes for me? *I tried to force them apart, but my outside wouldn't let them open.* Just try and relax now. You'll be just fine. *She patted my leg in assurance as she faded out.*

When I was finally able to breathe more normally, and because they had stopped checking on me, I ripped out the irritating nasal tubes. If I was stable enough to be left alone, I could breathe on my own, thank you. I lay there in bed awhile, incredulous at what had happened. This was definitely not the me I'd ever known.

Before I could move out of bed and get my head together, an aide whisked in with a wheelchair, announcing that I'd been scheduled for an emergency brain scan. What is this place?! I looked longingly at the bathroom as we raced by, out into the penetrating morning brightness of the hallway, my outside totally disheveled. Quite the sight as we wheeled past a group of gawking clinicians on rounds.

That's a private neurology patient, admitted last night from the ER.

Any Other Song

They smirked, mirroring knowing nods about the stereotypical neuro patient. I was numb to their sneers underneath my long scraggly hair, but inside—oh, I yelled and screamed at their cool detachment and cruel generalizations. I raged inside all the way down the elevator.

Is she a pediatric patient?

No. I'm trying to find Nuclear Medicine.

Oh, that's way back down the hall to your right, just past the elevators. *This had to be some kind of joke, parading me all over the outpatient corridor. I failed to see the humor in it. I crawled further inside from embarrassment, hoping no one could recognize my distorted outside that was groping for some hole to hide in. Then, barely noticed when I was finally wheeled into the lab, I was deserted.*

I thought of all the places I'd rather be than where I was, but settled for wishing I'd been able to just run a brush through my tangles. As that was impossible for the time being, I dreamed of sun-filled pines poking through powdery dust and pink granite, oozing with summer-warm midnights. I missed being at camp, lying on my bunk and gazing down the scrub oak hill to the lake, which was brilliantly blue at dawn; drinking in the twilight when the clouds were just orange wisps in the turquoise sky, the heat of summer afternoons lingering in the junipers and sage. . . . That's where I happened to fall for this tall tan lifeguard, and where I got my first dog bite, trying to break up the fighting watchdogs frustrated because they couldn't catch the prowler Ted never believed existed. What trust.

Are you Kathy? *No, I'm Athena in disguise!* Here. Drink this, and in half an hour we'll start the test. I know it doesn't taste too good, but you have to finish all of it. *She nearly witnessed projectile vomiting. Ichabod had promised this ordeal would only take an hour. Not that I had anything more pressing planned, but this wasn't exactly like any emergency procedure I'd ever heard of. Obviously nothing was really wrong or they wouldn't be taking so long. No big deal. So why hang around?*

When I was in sixth grade I remember roaring down the playground hill after this kid who'd doused me with water. It was after school and I wasn't supposed to be there anyway, let alone getting muddy, since the family was planning to go shopping after dinner. He went running under the swings, pushing one up as he darted through, the fireball in hot pursuit. I woke up face down in the gravel, blood oozing down my grimy face and slowly caking on

E. J. Daniel

my arm where my head had lain. *Fearful of what my father would say, I almost didn't go home. He exploded every time he had to pick up bits and pieces of his daughter. Another time, I was wandering around at the foot of a waterfall and someone must've heaved a rock off the cliff above. That time I woke up in the creek, several yards downstream, wet and bleeding. Getting to watch the doc sew me up was small compensation for my dad's icy silence. Since accidents continued to follow me into marriage, Ted often joked about trading me in for a new model, free of defects.*

Ok. We're ready for you. Lie down over here on the table, and we'll start the scan in half an hour or so. This will sting a little. *The hard cart was not conducive to withdrawal, and the shot hurt deep inside. I thought my head would explode.*

Hello. I'm Dr. Gaera. Mind if I have a look? *Why, help yourself. So nice to meet you. Sorry we couldn't be introduced under more desirable circumstances, but I'm sure you understand my predicament.*

All of my deeply imbued regimen in English called to mind relevant perspectives on cause and effect, and does the end ever justify the means, and what are the social ramifications of suicide in this novel? And what am I supposed to be learning from all of this shit, anyway, God?? What are You trying to tell me? Why can't I get the picture?

Ok, Kathy. Let me help you down. We need to have you sit in the chair over there by the drum. *This was too quickly evolving into a gothic nightmare of someone else's design.* Now, lay your head against this surface and hold it there. Good! *The technician began to strap my head to the huge steel-blue drum, so tightly I couldn't move if I'd had to. The two-inch straps forced me to stare into the cold, grooved surface, while the drone of computers in the small bright room numbed my throbbing head. I nearly collapsed to the floor when he unstrapped me.*

Now, turn your head to the right. *Anyone could be assured of one raging, uncontrollable headache after those Velcro bands were torn off and strapped on at so many different angles, strapping and unstrapping my head to the hum of the print-out results.*

> Attending note: brain scan negative. I still think she has early papilledema and have discussed arteriogram with Dr. Lister. We concur that it should be done to rule out posterior fossa or unusual hemispheric mass before doing the lumbar puncture.

Any Other Song

It was lunchtime when I was returned to the floor by a grungy orderly. My breakfast still waited for me, well-chilled. Before crawling into the fresh sheets, I staggered into the bathroom, barely acknowledging Ted as he walked in.

Where's Kathy? *So who's this voice?*

She's inside there. *More accurate than he intended.*

Well, we need to have her signature on this. Hope she hasn't eaten anything.

I held myself up over the sink, gazing into the mirror. They didn't need me to sign. I couldn't even make my name look like mine this morning to authorize the scan. Not that I had a choice in any of this. Too bad I couldn't just waste away into the walls. I gave up trying to make myself appear composed, venturing back into the room. Ted had disappeared. I plopped down on the edge of the bed, happy he'd bothered to stop in. Med school keeps 'em hopping!

Has she been prepped? *What was this green orderly doing standing near my bed with a stretcher? Why was he asking such a question of that nurse?*

No! You'll have to do it down there. *Then she helped him nudge me onto the cart. Too apathetic to protest, I was sort of relieved my case seemed to be getting more complicated, justifying my confusion. Tucked inside the blanket and railed snugly in, I fell asleep on the way down the yellow-tiled hall.*

Do you know what this procedure is, hon? *I slowly shook my head, thinking I might just take a rain-check on this one. The whole hospitalization was growing less and less enjoyable, even though intellectually it might have been interesting in a second person sort of way. That didn't change my sensation of being any ol' body shuffled from test to test.*

You're a little scared, aren't you? *At least the nurse was reading me right. Somebody ought to clue the docs in—soon.*

You want to give her a shot? They haven't even told her what we're going to do. *Her dusty blonde hair almost fell into my face as she leaned over to tell me I was going to get a shot to calm me down. She was easier to relate to than the motherly nurses on the ward.*

Hello. I'm the Head Nurse of Radiology. This will sting a little, but you should feel relaxed in just a little bit. There. *I had heard that one before, but I really hoped whatever was in it would dissipate the intense chills ravaging my strung-out body left alone in the institution-gray hall.*

The angio lab was surprisingly large, icy-green in its dimness.

E. J. Daniel

Outside, I was extremely lethargic, but my mind continued to reiterate endless "why"s.

She's going to have a general, isn't she?

No. And they didn't even prep her upstairs!

Those-in-green conversed as though I was already knocked out from the shot. Not that it didn't look that way, but I wished I could tell them otherwise. It was very uncomfortable having everyone standing around my flat outside as though I wasn't even there. The room was absolutely frigid, and being decked out for prepping didn't help my chills any. Half-awake I watched the staff gown each other up. Masked, gloved, and distant, they peered at me as I was immodestly soaped and shaved for the femoral puncture. They draped piles of sterile sheets onto me until the shivering finally subsided.

You're going to feel a little sting, now. *Normally I was stoic about shots and intrusive procedures, but my tolerance for pain seemed to be at a low ebb of late. That shot was supposed to locally numb the catheter entry site—and I was still waiting to feel the effect of the first shot.*

Do you know how to get a patient up on the table for shooting? *There must have been a new nurse on the team, so Honey showed her how to slide a patient up onto the table singlehandedly, grabbing me around my back, under my arms. She breezed me onto the x-ray table before I knew what had happened. Bravo!*

Hon, when they inject the dye through the catheter, you'll sort of feel a hot flash, but you need to lie very still so we can shoot the film. *My head nodded slowly, not comprehending exactly what a "hot flash" was, but it all sounded reasonable—and bearable. Not that I had a choice. The jab of the catheter stung where it entered the vessel, but it traveled unfelt inside while I watched its course on the videoscreen. Strange to see that little wire probing along, knowing it was inside me, and witnessing my own live x-ray like something out of a science fiction movie.*

Can you get into the right carotid? *One mask nodded as he twisted the catheter past the heart and into my neck. I was quickly losing any sense of curiosity in this procedure, having become very anxious about the location of the wire, and what it was going to do.*

Ok! We're there. *The triumphant mask nodded to Honey, who dropped into my consciousness like a bolt of lightning.*

Hon, we have to strap your head and chin down rather tight so you won't move while we take the pictures. *I realized this explanation*

19

Any Other Song

was more for my understanding than my consent, which had already been given by Ted. Nice of him to not stick around for the show.

My body stiffened in anticipation as she laid the straps across my forehead and chin, cranking them tight underneath, my head smashed into the padding. Then she taped my chin and neck, anchoring the ends to the table. And I completely understood the reason those-in-green went to all that trouble as soon as they flushed the catheter with the purple dye whose reservoir hung suspended like an IV bag next to the monitor. Suddenly it felt as though every vessel in my throat and mouth had exploded, the warmth of the hemorrhage gushing through my brain in foreign places, the rich aroma of blood flooding my mind. I thought my eyes were going to pop right out of their sockets as I wildly tried to tell anyone about the terrible mistake!

Hold still, now, hon. *She tried to restrain my arching body as the machine ricocheted under my head taking the cut films. Before the roar had stopped ringing inside, the fullness immediately faded from my head; but I was still tense, waiting, and wide awake.*

Alright. Let's pull out and do the left side. *They were sadists! Outside I was limp and slowly freezing to death, but the green mask was only interested in the cath, and Honey didn't seem to understand or hear my terror. Surely they wouldn't do it again. There had never in my life been a more terrifying nightmare than what was happening right then, and the distance between myself and what others saw outside only intensified my panic. I wondered if any one of those-in-green had gone through this personally, because no one could understand this until they've been there. The professional empathy failed to assuage my deepening horror and pain.*

How're ya doin', hon? Hold real still now! *She didn't read the fear inside, and my head blew apart again, bloody sensations saturating my brain. I tried desperately to run further inside to escape the tremendous shock, and the ricocheting dissolved into an empty silence. Those-in-green blurred somewhere else, and I didn't care anymore. I may as well have been dead.*

My god! Her hands and feet are like ice! *One of the nurses began massaging my fingers, which were poking out from under the sheet like sticks in a snow bank. Another nurse warmed my toe stubs between hands I couldn't feel. I needed to cry.*

Hey! What's happening here? You're breathing too fast. Slow down! *The green mask had wandered back in and seemed insensitive to my ballooning fear. I tried to hold my breath, to keep from cramp-*

ing into an unwanted rerun of my predawn ordeal, as the nurses continued to warm my frozen appendages. *She's too alert for having had all of that Valium. This shouldn't be happening.*

Did you see this? Those splotches weren't there a minute ago!

Honey had been watching the others attempt to salvage my outside when she must have noticed something on my throat, pulling down the neck of my hospital gown to further examine the rest of my chest. The green mask drifted over to see about the ruckus, while my body continued to mildly hyperventilate.

Get me some Benadryl! She's having a reaction! *The short, rotund manipulator jabbed a needle into my shoulder, my head still neatly bolted to the table. He left Honey to watch my outside as it slowly calmed.*

Is she alright now? They want to do a vertebral.

Hey—did you even get lunch?

No. I thought I'd try and sneak it in after we're through here. That new nurse can help out on the next case. I'm exhausted.

Are you going to eat downstairs?

Are you kidding? Eat that garbage? I'll just bike across the street.

In the snow?

My mind was slowly going from all the drugs that were finally taking effect, or else I was just tired from all the abuse I'd endured. The casual conversations assured me there was nothing to worry about.

Just one more time, hon. Hold real still again. *I'd been hoping they'd forgotten me. This time the hemorrhaging and ricocheting didn't even bother me—my senses were too dulled. Then they began to peel off all the tape that had held so wondrously.*

Let's get some help from next door to move her.

They've already gone to lunch.

Well. Then go on down to Radiology and find someone there, but we need some help.

Those-in-green heaved and hauled me back onto the stretcher, ushering me up to a strange floor. I hadn't even gotten to know my first roommate, except that she'd groaned incessantly all night.

A white blur was waiting in my new room, apparently to help spill my remnants into bed. It felt strange—all of those hands tugging to get me settled. A touching welcome to the neurology ward.

Can you get her over there?

Ready? Pull!

Really watch her. She's been on the pill for the last four years, and just had a reaction to the dye. *News travels fast.*

Any Other Song

The room was unbelievably glowing after the green dungeon. Sure, something exciting, sort of, had happened to me, but I was beginning to wish that I'd never said I'd had a headache. One by one the cloud of white thinned out, curtains drawn, lights turned out. A couple of nurses came back in to check on me, taking my temp and blood pressure as I lay immune to the outside. The lunch that had grown moldy waiting for me was removed.

> Radiology note: R-transfemoral angiogram. Patient had reaction to contrast (hives) which rapidly cleared with 50mg Benadryl. No other complications. Pulses intact. Both carotids and L-vertebral were studied. No aneurysms found, no mass lesions. Ventricles were normal.

CONSIDER

1. How could the physician translate to the patient his rationale for admission?
2. What kinds of patient education need to be initiated?
3. A functional nursing care plan for this patient would include what important problems and interventions?

THREE

> Attending note: patient feels bad with bifrontal headache and photophobia. Cerebral angiogram of all four vessels was within normal limits. R leg slightly cool, but not cold with good dorsalis pedis pulse. Best diagnosis is postviral encephalitis; doubt viral infection. Symptomatic control of headache, and watch and wait.

I was still tightly tucked and railed in bed on my new floor when sta-crumpled Bearl strolled in carrying a prep tray, a couple of student nurses trailing behind.

I need to do a spinal tap. Are you always so acutely brusque? The girls gingerly rolled me over onto my right side, holding me in that fetal position, while he took his time painting my back with betadyne. I'd always been curious about spinal taps. People say it's quite painful, but it couldn't be anything like a myelogram. The students were certainly more interested in all of this than I was.

This will sting a little, but you should feel better right away. That was a new one. I was just trying to figure out the rationale behind his declaration when slivers of pain shot up and down my back, into my legs and neck as he withdrew the fluid. This couldn't possibly make anyone feel better; he must have gotten his faulty info from the same place Honey had (just a "hot flash"). He dashed out with the syringe while the aspiring student nurses helped put me back

Any Other Song

together. What more could those-in-white cram in for one day before calling it quits?

Be sure you lie real still for a few hours, or you'll get a worse headache if you sit up. *And we don't want to endure that, do we? My smiling resident popped back to announce that all of my tests that day had been negative. So, I didn't have whatever they thought I had—whatever that was, since I was never told what those-in-white were looking for. So I was supposed to stand up and cheer for being negative? Terrific.* Actually, I was frustrated at not having something tangible to blame for the way I felt. But instead of retreating into the fog, my mind brewed a fire.

> Progress note: did lumbar puncture without difficulty. Patient tense. Fluid clear and colorless. Alertness, mental status the same. Follow for viral meningoencephalitis with supportive care.

It was consistently noisy but possibly convenient being in the room opposite the nurses' station, and at least I halfway kept up with all the goings-on in an otherwise dull entourage. Jo stopped by later that evening after I'd been burning for awhile. She tried visiting with me, but, restless with the heat, I just couldn't concentrate or appreciate her through my sweat. One of the more sensitive doctors-to-be, she felt my face and stuck the handy thermometer in my mouth. Affirmative action for my spreading apathy. When an aide motored into the room rationing out the evening water, Jo asked him to find his charge nurse STAT. Ted even drifted in at one point, but he seemed unable to say or do anything other than sit off to the side, either overly concerned or just being his usual preoccupied self. Maybe he and Jo could carry on a stimulating conversation together. I wasn't up to it.

A blonde cheerleader-type nurse bounced in apparently in response to Jo's request, studied the thermometer, noted my sopping-wet bed, the covers piled up at my feet. She said nothing but scurried out of my train of thought.

Call the resident! She's having another reaction. *Cheerleader roared back in, rolled me over and jabbed me with another needle. My body had too many invasions that day. Jo and Ted quietly excused themselves and I cried inside, feeling very used and misunderstood, frighteningly alone. I needed Jo to be there, just to sit or hold my hand, or something, even if I couldn't respond. I didn't know what was wrong with me, why I wasn't together, or even how to change where I was—or wasn't. Or whatever. In my mind I* *knew that God was probably there, somewhere, but it's nice having people around for tangible comfort. Reap "the rock" role, Kathy...*

> Note: called in to see patient, temp 38.6, hot all over with mild R groin pain. Patient did have reaction to angiogram this afternoon, and just after study, temp was 37.6. No infection, reaction to dye still continuing. Reevaluate in AM with CBC and differential.

What seemed like eons later my outside finally cooled down, but I laughed when I was only given aspirin for the raging in my head. All night I lay awake from fear of having another falling-out-of-bed sensation that might hurl me into hyperventilation. I was still temped, blood pressured and pupilled every 2 hours, which helped me stay awake, and I seemed to be slowly coming out of my distortion. If the doctors weren't finding anything, there was obviously no reason to stay in the hospital. It was too uncomfortable, the nights too long. Knowing everyone else was sleeping was eerie, and I just lay there, staring out the tall darkened windows at the few scattered stars still visible in the city. The incessant hum of the heating ducts must have finally lulled me to sleep.

I need to draw some blood. My, aren't we friendly this morning. Didn't get your morning coffee, huh? *The iceberg tech only drew a couple of tubes and I was relieved that's all I had to do with her. I got up, thinking I might try breakfast, but somehow it wasn't appetizing. Besides, I wasn't feeling too fresh and rested myself.*

Have you eaten? *That was not your I-am-concerned-that-you-didn't-eat question emanating from the curt orderly standing in the door with a stretcher. His green attire made me extremely uneasy, but I wasn't sure if it mattered, or if I just wanted it to matter. I was beginning to be wary of my outside, because of all the things it had tricked me into that I didn't need, since nothing was really wrong. At least I got to visit the bathroom first before he helped me crawl onto the token pad. Wrapping me up in more green, he jerked up the side rails and sped me down the brightly blurring halls to the elevators. My outside exited dizzier than before from the supine propulsion down the silent shaft.*

Have you ever had an electroencephalogram? *As I had been unable to be coherent that week, I just shook my head. At least, I hadn't had an official one. In our experimental psychology lab at college we used to play around with EEGs just to see who could get an alpha wave. I never did, but couldn't trust the machine anyhow.*

Any Other Song

This test won't hurt, I promise. Just relax, and if you feel like going to sleep, go ahead. *Falling asleep was the last thing I would let myself do; you don't just entrust your whole being to anyone, you know. All the lights were turned off except for a little glow in the corner where the console was and another lamp directly over my head so the tech could see where to goop up my scalp for the electrodes. Tedious work.* In a little while, this light will be flashing on and off. If it gets too uncomfortable, just say so. *I'd forgotten how long it had been since I'd been able to make intelligible conversation, emitting little more than a groan when it hurt too much inside. I wasn't sure what the strobe would do to me; it was frustrating that I wasn't more up on that. So much for the degree in psych.*

Ok. Open your eyes. *I could just make out the tech over in the corner, monitoring the procedure. It seemed like we were in some obscure cubbyhole in the bowels of the hospital, the room dark enough not to hurt. My inside felt more in control, so I could keep my eyes open.* Now close your eyes. *I was about ready to laugh this one off as a scientific joke when that light suddenly flashed on right in my face, making my whole body jerk with surprise, tense against the strobing brightness and abruptly ensuing darkness.* That's it! *Her perkiness made me feel like a total fool. She tried her best to swab up the blobs of jelly in my hair before sending me back upstairs. Hard to believe it's over. I mean, I wasn't even hurting—from the test, that is.*

> Progress note: patient feels less "spaced out" and her headache is somewhat better. Neck supple, right groin has minimal hematoma. EEG shows questionable, poorly developed alpha, but no asymmetry. Continue supportive care.

As I crawled into my freshly made bed, I noticed all of the flowers and plants crowding my half of the room. I nearly cried. It created a greenhouse out of the muddy-blue walled prison and I was thankful that something, at least, was thriving and alive. But I couldn't really appreciate the gestures of concern. No sooner had I collapsed under the covers than the neuro team rounded in. It felt as though I'd been a patient there a lot longer than two days.

Well, Kathy. All of your tests have been negative. *What else is new?* We're very pleased. You might just be able to go home tomorrow. *My, wasn't that fun? All those exciting tests just to find out what I didn't have, and still no one seemed to know what **was** wrong, but now that things are better, I can go home. Maybe I should've been* *grateful to Jo and Lindy for their prayers. God obviously had answered them by not letting anything be really wrong. So now it looked like I'd made it all up, which was totally unacceptable to me. Out of the question. Not me.*

Darley, Spence and Annie, my cohorts from the lab, interrupted the doctors, so those-in-white excused themselves amidst arms full of more flowers. Hey! You're making this place look like a morgue. *No one laughed.*

How're you feeling? You really scared us!

Scared you, Darley? Sort of better, but they still haven't told me what's wrong. Believe it or not, they said I might be able to go home tomorrow. Nurse Annie was thumbing through the chart at the foot of my bed.

Really? You don't look all that hot, though, I don't think. *What could I say? After a few minutes of nervous silence, they said goodbye, Annie reiterating how tired I looked. I knew my outside was a wreck, understanding they were just at a loss for words. It was Ok. I mean, what do you say?* Hey, thanks for coming up and bringing the flowers. *Darley started crying, so I didn't say anything else. As they turned to leave, I felt like a number one jerk for being the cause of someone else's hurt. I grew furious at myself for being where I was.*

Lunch and supper came and went, my head still too dull to absorb the intermittent attention being offered. I cringed to think about enduring another sleepless night interrupted by bed checks by the already overworked staff, but even those had become less frequent since I was no longer considered an acute case. I was going to be discharged the next day. Let's just call it all a big mistake, even though I knew those-in-white weren't sorry for all the grief they'd put me through. They figured it was a small blunder. Maybe I could still salvage part of the weekend, and pretend the nightmare had never happened. I didn't like being in a double bind: the docs wanted me there, but the nurses had better things to do than put out for someone who didn't need to be there in the first place. I felt guilty taking up a bed. Maybe they could move me down the hall into some corner until they could cheer my departure. Maybe if I fell asleep, it would be over sooner.

Hey! Know what I just found out? *It was 3:00 in the morning, and this RN was actually talking to me like I was a person. The room was still dusky dark except for the shaft of fluorescent light from the partially lit hallway.* We were born on the same day, the same year. I thought it was kinda neat! *Through her smile, she seemed like a*

Any Other Song

great person to know, mostly because she'd bothered to talk to me in the middle of a lonely night—even though she did wake me up. As Shannon strolled back into the brightness, her long brown hair hanging down past her waist, I wondered what it would be like to know her under different circumstances. What the hell was I doing here anyway? Almost all of the patients were much older than I, postcraniotomies or strokes, while the staff was my age. It was strangely funny to have my peers taking care of me, especially when nothing was really wrong. I wanted out of that place so bad. Outside, the snow began to fall past the large, gray windows.

> Progress note: patient more alert and less headache, but now weak. Generalized weakness of lower extremities with preservation of reflexes and sensation. Unable to walk by herself. Consider generalized weakness versus early Guillain-Barré!! Observe and ambulate.

During early morning rounds, which are always conducted during the patients' breakfast, I wasn't able to stand up alone and hop around for all those-in-white, who consequently ordered me back into bed for another day until, they said, they could be **sure** *I would be alright and that the virus wasn't progressing. Needless to say, I was simply thrilled to pieces. I gave up trying to outguess medical psyche, angry that my outside had failed to cooperate with the nice neurologists who were all dressed to go skiing after their Saturday morning duties. It seemed they just happened to stop by and see a couple of their patients on their way out of town. How considerate. After they'd left for bigger and better times, an understanding nurse came in to offer me a bath. I could handle anything but bedrest, so she helped me grope down the hall walls to the tub.*

I'll just kinda hang around to make sure you'll be Ok.

No really. Thanks. I'll be alright. *I could hardly wait to soap off the distasteful lingering remnants of those profoundly insightful tests, and allow myself to vegetate in bubbles. I didn't care enough to expend the necessary mental energy for heavy introspection.*

> Resident note: difficult problem—although headache is less severe, patient remains dull, apathetic and has clearcut significant proximal weakness of the legs with inability to stand on one foot without collapsing. Reflexes are preserved, cerebrospinal fluid protein was normal. She has truncal ataxia, but no clearcut sequential cord or brainstem signs. Fundi are unchanged with blurred discs and intact venous pulsations. She is afebrile with supple neck.

> Complains of parasthesia to touch right great toe. Etiology is uncertain, but I believe this patient is at risk to progress over the next few weeks to a profound organic brain syndrome and peripheral neuropathy. Consider Guillain-Barré, porphyria, vasculitis, but doubt cerebellar degeneration. Suggest EMG and nerve conduction.

The hours were melting by as snow continued to fall. I wouldn't have minded spending the day on the slopes, too. Shift after shift of nurses paraded through, and only if I stopped one of them did they ever converse at all with me. Not once had I put my idiot call-light on, and I never intended to. If nothing was apparently wrong with me, and no one took the time to tell me otherwise, then why should I bother the staff when they needed to tend to the potential fatalities biding their time up there.

> Attending note: agree with the chief resident—legs clearly weaker than on admission, no bladder/bowel symptoms. Some low back pain last night, but not now. Afebrile, fully alert, neck slightly tender. Probably seeing signs of hyalitis associated with the postviral encephalitis, but cannot rule out myopathy. Agree with muscular enzyme and porphyrin screen, cervical spine films, and watch and wait.

Me, myself and I were drifting. I wished I was nearer to the window, to stare at something other than pockmarked plaster walls and rotting spitwads on the bland ceiling. At least the last time someone slammed into a sterile tower, their rationale was obvious: get cut or go crippled. I remember lying in the basement two-bed ward crammed with four, my only view outside a mound of frozen dirt littered with molding autumn leaves. But it could have been worse.

That Saturday I should have done something productive with all of my free time, but I didn't care enough to bother, able only to bitterly rehash what I used to be able to do, say and feel. I'd already reached my prime, the climax ending abruptly with graduation—my reward: the privilege of helping hubby survive medical school. To rationalize my efforts his first year, I strove to be the submissive woman I thought he needed and wanted. But he spent even more time his second year buried deeper in his books, leaving me to entertain myself and laugh at all those people who continued saying, "Just wait! You'll be raking in the money soon enough." "You'll see—you'll end up compromising all those lofty

Any Other Song

ideals when you see how easy life'll be . . ." I think things would have been simpler and easier if he'd settled for being a science teacher or forest ranger in some western slope town, where I might have been able to find a job teaching, too. At least we'd be seeing each other, and talking. Wouldn't we, God? Or is this what you had in mind for us, for me? I'm impressed.

Not being able to really get away from everything used to make me feel like I'd literally crack up. I needed to have the sandstone bluffs and scrub oak to roam in during high school, away from the city and properly primped neighborhoods. Our dog would get so tired wandering around with me, I'd have to carry him home. I suppose one reason I kept going back to camp as a typically low-paid counselor was for my own catharsis, as though there was some magic hypnotic which the mountains exuded to pacify my subliminal self. I thrived on that tranquilizer. Probably my biggest mistake was substituting that necessary reality of needing to get away with the surrealism of a once-intimate relationship, transiently adequate at best. I understood later that was why I didn't care to see Ted. He simply had failed to understand me—if he had ever even taken the time out to try. Maybe medicine does that to people; maybe that's me finally seeing the real Ted.

> So brightly ripples the water
> in gentle rings of love
> once upon a yesterday
> and golden days are gone
> of laughter-woven
> heather haze
> shadowed dreams of
> warm emblazoned noons
> lemon
> in crimson, crackle
> rustling, yet soft
> twilight chills and
> moon silver-frosts
> columns of dying green
> so gentle dawn ribbons
> blue-shallow, and
> rainbows prism
> tomorrow's
> storm.

The aroma from the flowers grew more intense as nightfall drifted past, and I sought solace between the stark sheets and piles of open-weave blankets (the heavier the pile the cozier you feel). Everything else I simply forgot.

I was awakened by the most horrible stench as the woman beyond the always-drawn curtains lost all of her insides onto the floor. I tried to burrow back into oblivion, but the cleanup was just as noisy as the incident, and the male aide kept making grotesque faces which I found hysterical. After that I couldn't get back to sleep, and was awake when Shannon checked on me at 4 AM. I was anxious to visit, but instead of being met with the same compassion and smiles shared the night before, I encountered her well-drilled professionalism.

A 24-hour urine screen's been ordered on you, to begin immediately. Just store it in this bottle in the bathroom.

Wait! I'm supposed to go home today. Are you sure they meant it for me?

Quite! Doc's orders, so when you need to use the bathroom, call first. Sorry, Kathy. *She softened, but that didn't change my not going home. All black and white and never any gray. Ashes to ashes, dust to dust. And I bet that asinine test would be negative too. So, why bother? The game was getting old, and my attitude worse.*

> Progress note: patient says headaches and dizziness about the same, but more bright and alert today. Says weakness is improving and numbness on foot comes and goes. Fully alert, no back or neck tenderness. Normal muscle tone and active reflexes. Gait slow and unsteady, can't sit up out of chair unless on edge. Knee jerk asymmetry may be due to old ski injury to left knee. If patient has postinfluenza encephalopathy affecting white matter, it can logically affect the white matter of spinal cord. Plan to watch and wait.

Sunday slid by more comfortably, but I felt I'd been deserted by the doctors. Apparently we were out of the presumed crisis because no one came by the whole day to tell me what they failed to see on the spinal films taken that morning. But what did it matter? I just wanted out! Inside was finally winning over more of my outside, and a couple of the staff actually took time out to visit with me. Perhaps the more normal you appear, the more inclined they are to talk with you. A touch of positive reinforcement. Accepting the condition that if I was ever to get out of there I'd have to stay up, move around, and show everyone I was "just fine," I staggered

Any Other Song

down the hall to the showers—alone. To finish what I didn't quite succeed at Saturday in getting rid of the test particles.

The afternoon was a frozen, snowy gray when Ted dropped by to help me stroll around the floor, past the room where the policeman sat guarding the critically ill prisoner who'd tried to assault one of the nurses last night. We made note of the revamped north wing, completely carpeted and padded, where the adolescent psych ward would soon move. It was appropriately located on the same floor as neurology. Beyond the drapeless windows at the far end of the wing snow continued to fall, blanketing the concrete in subtle softness. Ted became bored aimlessly wandering around the halls with his degenerate wife, trying to keep me steady as he returned me to the greenhouse. *Catch ya later.*

Fantasizing someone would make note of it in my chart, I offered to escort my excised-brain-tumor roommate down the hall to the TV room. I was tired of her complaining about how none of the nurses ever took any time off to walk her around the halls. As we gimped along the wall, Cheerleader breezed by all perfumed, smiling proudly at our grand effort. What a pathetic picture we must've painted. But my partner proved too ill to stay and watch the movie, so I let her stagger back to the room alone. I sort of hoped someone would come to check on me or something. As the hours crawled by, for all they knew, I could've crunched.

The large, sparsely furnished room was dark except for the hazy light of the television screen. I thought I was alone until I heard some movement in the back of the room, and when I turned to look I saw a couple of white eyes staring at me. I quickly turned around to pretend I was engrossed in the movie, but could only think about all the recent reports of rape. What if he tried to go after me? No one was around on Sunday night, and it'd be me and him in the shadowy, single-entrance room. I might not be found for hours, and could be close to dying before I would be missed. There was no way I could fight. Suddenly he hopped up from the stacked chairs in the back, and I tensed for whatever, still pretending to watch the screen, as he walked toward the hall.

Did you get dinner?

Yeah. Downstairs. Still have to finish cleaning 7 East. Real slow tonight. His partner moved on to the freight elevators.

What a story that'd make—"Neurology Patient Attacked by Janitor. A 23-year-old patient of the medical center hospital was molested by an off-duty housekeeper Sunday night, and nursing staff failed to discover the victim until several hours after the alleged incident." Maybe then I'd have cause to be an inpatient.

 He sauntered back in the room, plopping down on a couch directly across from me. I kept my eyes glued to "McMillan & Wife," but he'd blown my concentration. His close proximity made me ridiculously nervous, and finally fear won over my sordid sense of adventure. I excused myself at a commercial and rocketed out of the lounge, weaving back into my room unnoticed. Too tense to sleep, I pulled a chair from the room into the doorway to watch the world go by. The policeman was making small talk with some of the staff at the nurses' station, and when he saw me he decided to saunter over. Lucky me.

 Hi there. Slow night, huh?

 For sure. How long are your shifts?

 Oh, me and another guy moonlight on this one for 12-hour spells. Patient's a real jerk. Keeps pulling out all of his tubes just to get one of them nurses in there. They have to keep him real sedated so he won't try nothin'. *Wonderful. I can't remember the rest of the small talk, since my mind was someplace else. I'd rather have been talking to Shannon. Or Jo. He said "so long" soon to retake his vigil outside his prisoner's room. I got tired of trying to function normally, and retreated to bed. Just as I dozed off, an incredible crash jolted me awake.*

 Shit! You won't believe what happened! *Out in the hall the nurses were in an uproar.* The TV just fell on top of this guy down in 7228. *That sent me into hysterics. What a circus! Finally, I was laughing at something, and laughed at myself for laughing. Maybe I was Ok after all.*

 We've sent him down to the ER for an x-ray. He's probably got a skull fracture with our luck.

 So how did it happen? It just fell?

 Would you believe he was trying to actually steal the TV right off the wall? *And this was supposed to be a haven of convalescence?*

FOUR

I'm really sorry, but I just can't let you go home today. Your legs aren't strong enough, and . . .

I couldn't believe that Bearl had the gall to tell me such a terrible thing, and outside I sighed him to silence. Just so I'd be able to go home I'd been up early, walking, moving around. I was even in a decent mood before he'd come in. I'd tried. I had really tried and then he dared to tell me no-go in that shallow manner of those-in-white. I was enraged at this whole cruel game—God included; I just wasn't learning the rules fast enough to keep up and get out. Screw everyone, because I quit!

> Progress note: patient feels better but careful questioning revealed headache still present but intermittent. Exam essentially unchanged from yesterday. C-spine film within normal limits. Blood drawn. Plan to observe.

Dull, dull, dull. Breakfast was typically bland and left uneaten. Why should I stuff my face anyway? All I did was lie around all day. Mentally dulled, I plodded down the hall for my morning shower, ending up in the tub since I didn't have the energy to withstand the energetic water. Besides, soaking takes more time and maybe the day would go faster. When I wandered back into my

Any Other Song

room, the curtains were all open, the sun reflecting brilliantly off the snow-covered outside, making my bed almost glow. But the cheeriness only exacerbated my irritability. A stereotypical Monday morning, the staff was too busy to talk away my boredom, so to maintain my patient image, I went to bed. Occasional visitors paraded through, pitying expressions as though saying "what can I do to help?" Nothing, unless you'd like to trade places with me. My outside was being downright bitchy, but even I couldn't find anything to crack a smile over. I'd really been counting on going home and forgetting that all of this had happened. Playing sick when I didn't know why I should be wasn't my best role. And no answer came when I demanded "why?" of the God I couldn't find anymore.

And the suffocating cloud drifted back to further flatten my distorted affect, just when one of Ted's friends was attempting to converse with me. I thought it terribly coincidental that I should be getting worse in her presence, as though she could subtly obliterate me. With me out of the way, she could have Ted to herself; he'd be happy. At first I tried to fight it off, but gave up half out of curiosity. Maybe I wouldn't be bothered then. I didn't even see her leave.

> Nursing notes: patient hesitant to admit discomfort. Complained of numbness in left leg and one episode of dizziness. Afebrile. Anxious to go home.

The big, Swedish-type nurse who'd helped me shower last week bothered to stay awhile and talk. She was one of the more empathetic of the staff since she didn't come across harried, as though the entire floor would stop functioning if she lingered too long. But I still felt like a Venus flytrap for wanting her to stay. I've been trying not to be a bother, you being so busy and all, but it's getting a little boring for me.

Oh—I know we don't spend enough time with the patients that aren't as sick as some of the others. In report, everyone says what a good patient you are, since you never call anyone. I suppose that's sort of a poor way to look at it, but we're just so busy with some of our terminal patients. Being understaffed doesn't help any, either, but— that's just our excuse. We really should be spending more time with you.

Maybe. It's just hard being right across from the nurses' station, 'cuz I'd rather be out there with anyone, than lying here in bed!

I guess I would, too. Well, I'd better get moving, but I'll talk to you later. You seem dizzy, so I'm putting your side rails up. Ok?

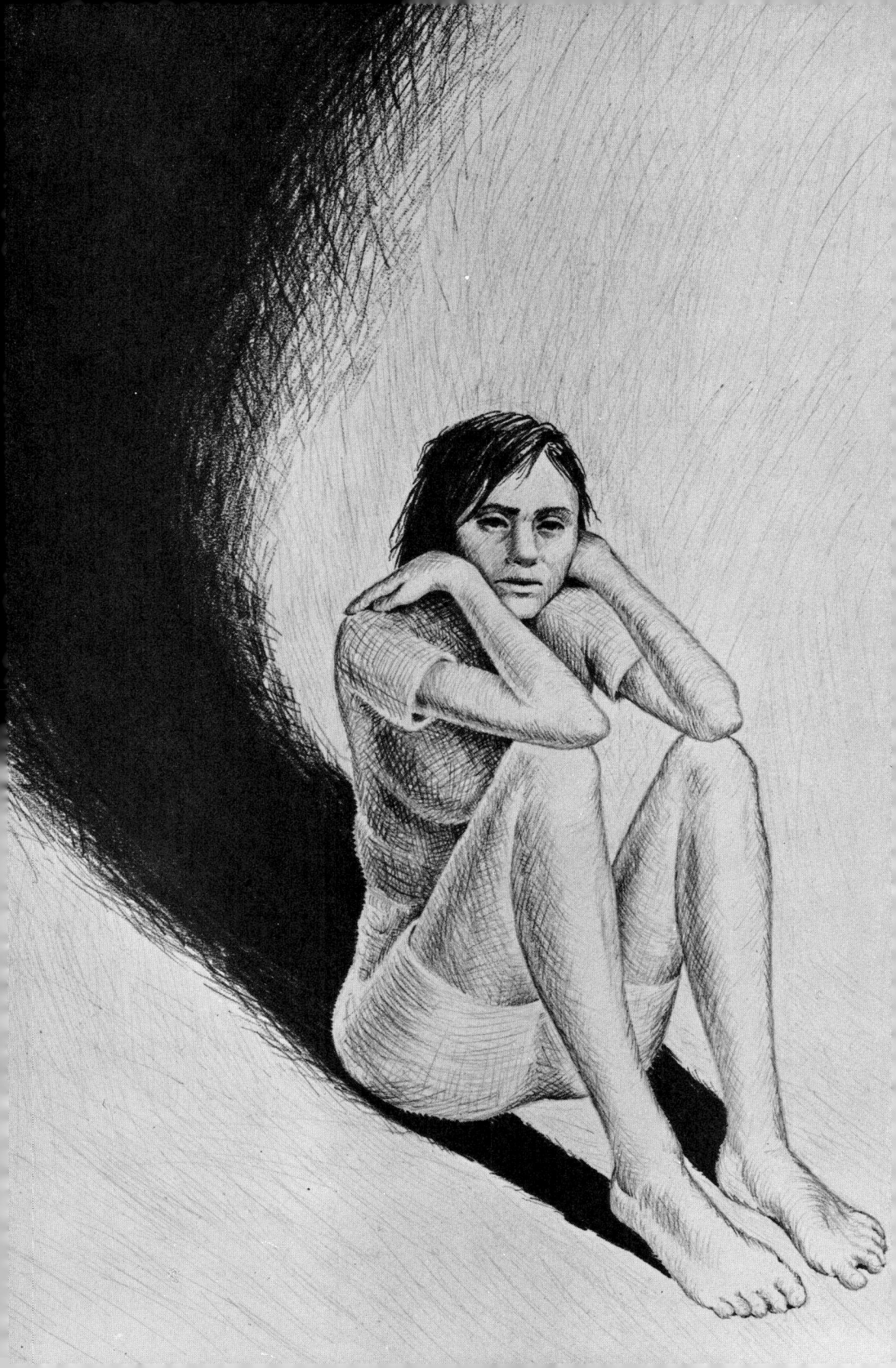

E. J. Daniel

I really felt guilty letting her take care of me, feeling stupid and uncomfortable being the patient. It would've been alright, though, if the roles had been reversed. I can handle that without feeling put out or anything. But I never could feel justified letting someone care for me—that was too much to ask. Too demanding. And not worth it.

Jo stopped by later during the afternoon, mostly sitting idly by the bed, making small conversation while I mumbled back some incoherent response. It was great just having her there, and I hoped she wasn't growing angry at my uncooperative outside.

When the evening shift of nurses rounded through before report, a frosty-haired RN bent over my bed. Hi Kathy. How're you doing?

She was so genuinely warm that, out of surprise, I failed to reply. Jo greeted her for me. You don't know BJ? *I shook my head.* She's a really neat Christian. *That much I heard, before withdrawing to think about some other time. I couldn't blame Jo for giving up finally, and leaving. I wasn't exactly a joy to be around and couldn't fully appreciate the time she gave up to spend with me. To escape the bright light filtering in through the windows, I closed my eyes.*

> *It was especially foggy that morning—the air heavy with damp, chilling mist, the sand hard-packed and gray. The frothy green waves crashed onto the beach—roaring and pounding—evoking all the feelings I'd been repressing for so long. Spray from the surf stung my face, while the gulls screamed.*

Kathy, are you feeling alright? *Dusk had finally beaten the afternoon. Inside I was trying desperately to keep it together, but BJ seemed to know it wasn't working. Finally someone was seeing inside me, and I trusted her as I hadn't been able to trust anyone else. I felt an odd sense of relief that she was there, but the cloud got heavier and darker, and I couldn't stop myself from spinning around the muddy room. I was losing, and I panicked.*

BJ came back in with a narcotic for my incessant headache since the placebo aspirin failed to take effect. Maybe after that I wouldn't feel the hurt or have to face the impending nightmare. I didn't understand why the cloud was making it harder for me to breathe.

Um. I don't think I'm feeling my right foot, or can't move it. *BJ stopped at the end of my bed and uncovered the frozen toes, looking curiously at me.* It's probably just an hysterical reaction or something. It's Ok. *I realized too late how that must have sounded and couldn't believe I'd let that sorry explanation pop out, practically a confession that none of it was real—that it was all in my head afterall, and not organic. I felt betrayed! I couldn't imagine what

Any Other Song

was happening. My outside seemed to have taken over (or what I thought was my outside, because I didn't know that part of me). Not any more. My body kicked into a blasting hyperventilation attack. It felt like something was trying to suffocate me, and I was completely out of control.

Kathy! Are you having trouble breathing? BJ had come back in with the familiar green tubes, noticed my gasping, and hooked me up as the intern, who'd followed her into the room, jabbed a catheter into my left arm to draw blood.

The room dimmed, and I realized I'd drifted through a sunset-turned-midnight. BJ took my cold, cramping hand in hers; in her warmth, I blurted out that I'd heard she was a Christian. She just looked at me funny. The oxygen wasn't helping at all, and I tried to tell them that I just couldn't get enough air, but my eyes wouldn't open to warn of my terror. Then the intern yanked my eyelids open, flashed a light in my face to look inside, but couldn't find me. He plunged a needle deep in my right wrist, which didn't help my fear. Everyone seemed to be rushing around, shouting orders, and I ran further away to watch. Then I noticed my pastor standing in a corner of the room, praying. Jesus! What is going on here?

Get a bed down in Intensive! Suddenly my bed was pulled away from the wall, into the middle of the small, curtained-off half of the room. They had unplugged the oxygen, fumbling to set up the portable oxygen. My body was heaving and gasping, cramped up in pain.

Those-in-white were outside in the hall consulting when I stopped breathing. I thought it incredible that I could be quietly lying there, awake inside, while my outside refused to breathe. It felt like I didn't need to, so why bother? I was too tired anyway, and it was nice being able to finally lie still, totally relaxed and flaccid. I told the Lord that apparently I was dying, and if that's what He wanted, who was I to argue? I was just relieved it was finally over.

Uhm. Hey, anyone! She stopped breathing—about a half minute ago. I'd been wondering if the aide standing beside my bed was going to notice or just appreciate the pleasant silence along with me.

I was nearly unconscious when the intern roared back in, shoved the aide aside and smashed his knuckles into my chest. *That* was certainly more breath-taking than inflating. *Flush her with oxygen! Get that tank over here and hook her up!* A black mask was plopped over my face and I was smothered with a blast of air. That didn't give them their desired response. *Someone get the elevator!*

E. J. Daniel

As the intern dug his knuckles into my chest again, I gasped in deep pain. Kathy! Open your eyes! Kathy, c'mon! Breathe! Open your eyes! *He kept yelling at me, and when I couldn't respond, grinded my chest again, over and over until I gasped out a couple of shallow breaths. The portable tank and mask were too bulky to fit, so they discarded it. While we raced down the hallway to the elevators, my outside, coaxed and grinded, obligingly spit out occasional breaths. Inside I was willing to cooperate, even though it looked like it was all over, but I honestly had no control.*

Crammed inside the stainless steel elevator, I vaguely perceived BJ standing at the foot of my bed, her eyes wide but caring. I was putting too many people out again, and I was really sorry it had all happened, sorry for all the trouble it was causing. They should have just let me go . . .

The elevator screamed to a halt, spitting us out into another hallway. The team hauled me from my bed onto a stretcher, and rushed me into the Intensive Therapy Unit. As I was whisked from the cart onto the narrow IT bed, I could see BJ sitting nearby, writing furiously in my chart. My flannel gown was pulled off my body, abruptly ending any modesty, and all those-in-white crowded around to listen with their stethoscopes. They pulled me from side to side, while the nurses hurried to plug me into their monitors.

During a break in the furor, BJ came over to the bed. Kathy, the nurses here can take better care of you. That's why we moved you down here. *Gingerly she patted my IV arm and left. Inside I begged for her understanding, crying at her desertion, not caring any more about anything. I was cuffed for blood pressure and ordered to move this leg, now the other, open your eyes, lift your arm. Go away . . .*

> Nursing notes: gave p.o. med and almost immediately patient was unable to move right toes. Began hyperventilating and simultaneously or slightly after began contracting both hands and wrists in decorticate manner with pain in hands. Responded appropriately to questions. Just before transfer to IT, became lethargic and difficult to arouse and apneic for 20–30 seconds. BP 122/110; 130/92, respirations 154, pulse 116–130. Transferred to 6N.

I couldn't perform very well for those-in-white. Since I wasn't really there, it didn't matter what any of them did to me.

She looks peaceful now. That strange new doc didn't know I was dead as he stood at the foot of my naked body.

Well, she doesn't have a pulmonary embolism. *Dr. Bearl had been*

Any Other Song

going over me with mechanical precision.

What about a metabolic disorder? *The intern was immediately silenced by Bearl's glare. Dr. Dobber motioned everyone out into the hallway as he removed his stethoscope.*

The nurses quickly tucked me into bed, then braided my scraggled hair—IV still running, arm still cuffed, rectal thermometer still in place. A third nurse returned from the conference outside.

You mean all of this is psychological? *Those two sounded surprised; I was stunned! It was impossible! To stay another damn night was Bearl's idea, not mine!* They *had ordered it all. Just because those-in-white couldn't find something drastically, obviously wrong was no cause to proclaim to the entire hospital that it was all in my head!*

Oh, no! I forgot her thermometer! *The pigtailed RN tried to stifle her laughter. Real funny.*

They said it's sort of a fugue state she's in now. *They carried on as though I couldn't hear them. This was more than I could bear.*

Inside, I tried to sort everything out. After all, I was an intelligent, together person—once upon a time—and this could all be explained rationally. I knew myself well enough, I thought, to know that it couldn't be merely psychological. Surely someone would see that the virus had made me someone I wasn't. It was only logical.

> Progress note: patient developed the sudden onset of hyperpnea, weakness and frenzied posturing of her wrists. Had been feeling weaker all afternoon, but was up and about earlier today. Now peaceful and calm, speaks in unisyllable, short phrases. Discs are flat. Wiggles fingers right and left, toes left only. Reflexes brisk, toes decreased. No edema. Feels pin prick in all extremities. This is a rather difficult case. I've never seen a clinical picture like this. Could be acute anxiety versus a myelopathy. Recommended repeat lumbar puncture.

I kept turning over in my mind all of the possible different explanations for what had happened, wondering if I really did know myself. The oxygen continued to hiss in my nose, while one of the monitors beeped softly from the wall.

> Nursing: 23-year-old female transferred from 7W. Admitted to hospital for headache workup. All tests within normal limits. Cold right leg and bilateral tingling of legs and inability to move right toes, began to hyperventilate and became decorticate with 10–15 sec. periods of apnea. Upon unit admission, patient very lethargic,

disconjugate eye movements, pupils dilated. Muscle spasms without involving trunk. Simple withdrawal to pain, moves only to command. Oriented, BP 142/90, pulse 90, respirations 12 with apneic periods.

I was fighting to open my eyes, when it suddenly occurred to me that it wasn't me that was trying to suffocate myself, but something else. It sounded really crazy, but I couldn't think of any better answer—I was under Satanic attack! How should I know why he would pick on me? Why did anyone freak out? Who knows? It scared me to think that might've been the answer, especially since there was no way in the world I could ever explain it to the docs. You know how that goes. But denying that it could exist doesn't mean it absolutely can't. So, in Jesus' name, I commanded Satan to be gone—and my eyes jerked open. Scared to death, I let out a long, slow breath.

Hey! She's awake! *I just laid there staring up at the ceiling, terrified. That kind of answered prayer I'd never experienced, and the implications I couldn't begin to imagine.*

Pigtails hurried over to the side of my bed and smiled. How're you feeling?

I turned my head toward her, hoping desperately she would see how frightened I was. But how could she know what was going on inside? Is it too late to call that nurse upstairs that helped transfer me down? I really need to talk to her.

Oh. Well, sure. What's her name? *She seemed kind of put off that I'd asked for BJ, but called upstairs anyway.*

She'll be down as soon as she finishes report. Ok? *I nodded, thanked her profusely, and settled back to wait. The nurses in the unit weren't too talkative either, preoccupied as they were with watching all their monitors. I concentrated on the clock, attempting to maintain control.*

Progress: patient began moving spontaneously, awake, alert, talking easily. Stable, feeling weak. Attending aware of increased level of consciousness. Observe.

Hey! How're you doing? *Familiar question, familiar welcome voice. Now that I was more together, I was surprised at how good it felt to see her, but the fear prevented me from reaching out.*

What do you know about the supernatural? I mean, is it possible that what happened to me tonight, could be explained that way? *She seemed naturally surprised at first, but then must have understood the remark I'd made earlier to her. I needed an answer!*

She looked at me intently. Kathy. I think, medically, that the cere-

Any Other Song

bral swelling could probably alter your mind enough so that you might be susceptible to that kind of full-blown anxiety attack. As Christians, though, I don't believe the Lord would allow Satan, if that's what you mean, to possess us. But I do suppose there could have been enough physiological changes to allow this to happen to you. Does that make sense? *I nodded, staring back up at the ceiling.*

I knew I must be sounding terribly irrational and very unmedical, and probably no one would ever really know or understand what had happened to me. But at that time, I was content to be awake, and relatively calm. The beeping was endless.

Tell you what! I'll try and explain this to your attending, if I get a chance. I've got to get back to my floor now, but I'll leave my home phone with the nurses here in case you need to call. Ok? *BJ smiled warmly, squeezing my arm in assurance. I felt I didn't deserve to know such an understanding and concerned person. She hurried out, after leaving her number scribbled on a yellow pad, and as she disappeared through the door, so did my alertness. Maybe I was just tired after the ordeal. I floated off into an eerie twilight.*

> Nursing: patient stable, afebrile; increased alertness noted throughout shift. Moving all extremities on command and spontaneously. Oriented to time, place and recent events. During deep sleep some slight twitching of right hand and thigh noted. Continue to observe.

Those-in-white, without my attending, came early Tuesday morning, but not before the predawn bath given to the lady next to me. The bath made even more noise than the wheezing asthmatic they'd admitted earlier. My IV had been pulled, the oxygen unplugged, the monitor unhooked. They'd cranked me up in bed so I could stare at my breakfast. The nurse, trying to help me reorganize myself, left when the docs trotted in. Seeing Bearl made me ill.

You realize, Kathy, that it's your own fault now that we have to keep you here another couple of days. Otherwise you could have gone home. *He had to be kidding! But as I looked from face to face, I realized how very serious the neuro team was about it all being strictly psychological. You lose, Kath. . . .*

I started crying, which probably only confirmed their diagnosis, and they uncomfortably backed out of the curtained cubicle. The nurses couldn't help overhearing, and one brought me some Kleenex.

You know, you really should try and eat something.

I can't eat. *She stood there, not knowing what else to say to me. At least the nurses gave a shit.*

Dr. Forster himself interrupted her compassion, closing off the curtains behind her. He sat down, rather fatherly, on the edge of my bed. What happened?

As I tried to explain away Bearl's accusation, I started crying again, relating how I was really awake inside the entire time, hearing everything, trying to cooperate with them, but nobody was understanding, jumping to all kinds of crazy conclusions and never telling me anything.

Ok, Ok! Just calm down, now. We'll go ahead and send you home today, if you promise to come in and see me in the clinic early next week. I'll straighten things out with the other doctors, and you can just see me. How does that sound? *In his beard and thick glasses, he appeared very Freudian—concluding we had come to some kind of an understanding of the whole situation.* Give me a call on Friday to tell me how you're doing. *He smiled and exited through the curtains. I sat staring in disbelief at the floor, wondering if BJ had succeeded in talking to him.*

The nurses pulled back the curtains, ready to transfer me out. Kathy, they're waiting for you back upstairs.

Could you hand me that yellow slip of paper with the phone number on it?

Sure. Are you ready to go? *Quite.*

When I arrived upstairs, the staff seemed happy to see me in one piece, I guess because I'd probably given them all a good scare. My bed was made, lunch ordered, and the curtains opened out onto the melting snow. I got dressed in anticipation of leaving, lying in bed until Ted could get there to take me home. It was all so cheery, bright and hustle-bustle, as though last night had never happened . . .

> Discharge note: patient was an ill, slow-moving girl. Recent, remote and immediate recall were intact. There was a good fund of knowledge. She was frightened and could not concentrate well, somewhat stoic. The patient could hear well. It was felt that the episode of hyperventilation was anxiety-related. Apparently, the patient had some difficulty being in the hospital and did not like being here with acutely ill patients. She had difficulty recognizing that she had an anxiety reaction, and felt that something else was wrong. The patient is being discharged with a final diagnosis of post-influenza encephalopathy and possible associated myopathy. She will be continued on aspirin prn for her headaches. Some discussion with the husband revealed that the patient seems to have had some

Any Other Song

problem arise prior to some of his exams, and this will be looked into further.

> *i remember*
> *sometime*
> *in a yesterday*
> *when i used to*
> *crave getting away,*
> *alone, anywhere,*
> *just to know again*
> *who i was*
> *and why.*
> *Then someone entered*
> *that lonely place*
> *to live a loving cause for being*
> *and growing*
> *together. But something*
> *shattered*
> *making me some pawn*
> *of any other's ego*
> *and surviving alone has become*
> *my sunflower fugue. And i*
> *laugh*
> *at what you call healing*
> *as you suicidally destroy*
> *each other all in the name of*
> *medicine.*

CONSIDER

1. According to Harrison's *Principles of Internal Medicine,* encephalitis is defined as " . . . an acute febrile illness with convulsions, stupor or coma; aphasia or mutism; ataxia. . . . Diagnosis is dependent on demonstrating focal derangement of function of the cerebrum, brainstem or cerebellum. In patients with viral encephalitis, there is a 5–20% mortality." What specific behaviors and rationale exhibited by the patient support this diagnosis?
2. In terms of accuracy and completeness, how representative of the patient's observations and feelings are the various medical notes?

---

*Harrison, *Principles of Internal Medicine,* 8th Edition, McGraw-Hill, 1977, pp. 1897-1899.

FIVE

After those-in-white let me out of the white-tiled mecca, I tried to recuperate for a few days in an attempt to find me again, pretending the hospitalization had just been a mistake. Everything was going to be alright, and I could just sort of forget it had even happened. But it didn't work out that way. Inside, I was too tense, too scattered, and too out of control.

Ted called Dr. Forster a few days postdischarge regarding my continued dizzy spells. I'd even blanked out long enough on the telephone for my sister to have noticed; she finally brought me back by shouting. But Forster thought the spells and the eye-blurring were strictly anxiety related. I wasn't looking forward to seeing him in clinic after that.

Monday I showed up in clinic to see Dr. Forster. In response to his absurd allusions regarding possible marital difficulties, job-related anxiety and dissatisfaction, I became extremely reserved and vowed not to return for follow-up. He put me on Valium to try and calm my increasing lack of composure. Arriving home, I took my pills like a good girl, strolled upstairs and parked my body on the carpeted floor in a corner of the spare bedroom. When Ted came home from class, the lights were out, dinner wasn't ready, and he stormed upstairs wanting to know what was wrong.

I just want to be left alone.

Any Other Song

Why do you have the lights out?
It hurts my eyes.
Do you want to talk?
No, I said! Now just leave me alone! Please!
I'm gonna call Jo.
I don't care what you do. Just leave me alone! *Ted went into the other room, and I could just barely hear him talking to someone. The night before, when I'd been talking with Lindy, I felt like I was slowly losing my mind, and couldn't remember things. I didn't know what was wrong. Maybe I was angry at God for not letting everything be alright since it was supposed to be over and done with. Lindy didn't seem to know what to say to ease my anxiety, and I concluded I shouldn't have been dumping on her anyway—but I felt desperate for help.*

Jo's coming over. *Ted frowned at me, justifiably frustrated at his crazy wife, and clumped downstairs.*

> Clinic note: subject feeling fairly well—occasional headaches relieved by aspirin. Main problem is "dizziness" and unsteadiness, especially on exercising or arising. No falls. One episode of talking on phone when she "blacked out" for 20–30 seconds, but without fall or slump, just without responding to other person. She is alert, discs the same. Still a difficult diagnosis. Residual effects of encephalopathy versus anxiety and hyperventilation. Discussed my ideas and psychological issues. Valium 2mg t.i.d. Decide later on prognosis.

I was on the ski slopes, flying down the mountain, everything clean and white. But I couldn't go fast enough. Nothing was going fast enough. Patience wasn't one of my qualities.

Kathy! What are you doing? *Jo suddenly appeared. Maybe I really did want someone to come over, to show me they cared about me. It wasn't enough to believe that God was somewhere around.*

I don't know. *I was sure she thought I was behaving like a lunatic.* I feel drunk, but I've only had my Valium. I'm dizzy, slow, confused; I keep having hyperventilation spells, my eyes blur. I don't know what's wrong. *But it seemed appropriate for me to be sitting on the floor, coiled in the darkness.*

Ted had followed Jo upstairs, but she closed the door on him and turned on a dim light in the opposite corner of the small, cluttered study. I was amazed at how gently Jo was handling my derangement. I'd always been reticent to open up to her because she always seemed to have all the answers (except the one summer when I'd had alternatives for her). But she was strong enough to fight it off then, and carried on stronger than ever. What Jo shared with me I can't remember, but she slowly helped draw me out of my distance, so that I could keep on trying.

By Wednesday, my resolve not to see Dr. Forster was even stronger. If I had made myself ill, I could just as easily make myself well, and he was mistaken in thinking there was something wrong with my marriage just because he'd had trouble in his when he was in medical school. I wasn't known to be the kind of person in dire need of psychiatric care—as he'd implied—and I was determined to resolve this all myself. Mom always said I could do anything if I wanted to badly enough. Besides, my dog decided to deliver her puppies the morning of my clinic appointment, so I hastily wrote a letter to Dr. Forster and asked Ted to deliver it to him.

> I hope you forgive me for not showing up for my second appointment. As long as there is still some question of my symptomatology being "psychological," I see no reason to be seen in your clinic.
>
> I know that wives of medical students and doctors go through a great deal, and even have a notorious reputation for manifesting "unusual" symptoms. I apologize for being rather incensed about the possibility of my episodes even being due to anxiety. Feel free to talk with anyone who really knows me as to whether that's plausible.
>
> I discontinued the Valium yesterday, and if there is some medical/clinical basis for my symptoms, they will probably emerge later. Otherwise, I thank you for your excellent care, your fatherly concern, and the fascinating glimpse into neurology.

On Friday of my first full week back at my two jobs, a big ten days since I'd been out of the hospital. Darley, Spence and I decided to hit FAC because it'd been such a rotten day. As I was feeling zero effect from the tranquilizers I was taking prn, I didn't think twice about gulping down the five Harvey Wallbangers in an hour and a half. I always enjoyed drinking with Darley since she was genuinely friendly and even sisterly toward me.

You know, Kathy, you're alright. But you shouldn't have mixed it up. *Darley seemed as drunk as I was, but insisted on driving me home. It all seemed hysterically funny at the time, but Ted wasn't laughing with us when I rolled into our apartment hanging between Spence and Darley, several hours late from work. I figured he wouldn't even notice since he had so many books to keep him company. No big deal.*

Any Other Song

When I woke up Wednesday morning thinking it was Saturday, I should have known things wouldn't go well and stayed home to nurse the pups. In the school lounge before class began, I got in on the climax of a heated conversation between the principal and a teacher over a letter she wanted to send to a student's parents. He was suppose to read it first "to edit it" (meaning to censor it). Mr. G strutted out, leaving her fuming over her coffee. As the teachers left to round up their kids, I lingered awhile over my hot chocolate. Suddenly Mr. G burst back into the lounge, demanding to know why I had spent an entire afternoon alone with one of my counselees the day before. His explosive entrance caught me by surprise. En garde!

Mr. G! I thought it was better to keep Dan in my room and try to calm him down, rather than leave him stewing out in the front office. There was quite a collision between Dan and his teacher, and I wanted him to understand how he could have averted the blowup in class.

Is that all you did? He sounded incredulous, and continued fingering all of the old cigarette butts in the ashtrays—to get tobacco for his pipe.

The remainder of the time he sat in my office doing his homework. *He snorted at that explanation and lumbered out, plowing his way through the hyperactive students.*

Later that morning I telephoned the school psychologist for some follow-up concerning the visit he agreed I should have with the mother of one of my students. Little had been accomplished because she had babbled on for 45 minutes about everything but her son's school problems. The kid's teacher, who shared my disgust for the way the schools were operating under Title I, was anxious to make any progress with him. At 12:10, this kid's mom called me, unbelievably upset, demanding that I come over to her house "right away!" I said I'd try, but that I needed to get over to my other school. I grew quite uneasy about her call, fearing that it involved a letter I'd mailed out "uncensored"—which had probably backfired. Before I could get back to her, my supervisor informed me that it was not my place to "talk religion." It was a parochial school and all I'd done was answer a few simple questions asked by my students.

Also, young lady, it's not your place to recommend that any of these students transfer back into a public school . . . *regardless of the fact that one of the kids wanted to and her parents were in agreement . . .* And your mere presence has caused a lot of grief among the entire faculty here! *Bingo, Kathy! Wonderful testimony you've given.*

Ok. I'll hash it out with all of the involved teachers tomorrow over lunch. Ok? Then I'll talk to the parents again about the transfer. Ok? Now, I'll just shut up. *What a lesson in humility—and I hadn't even prayed for it. Before I had a chance to regroup, I was informed that Mr. G wanted to see me immediately. Bad vibes, and good-bye.*

As I'd suspected, the mom was upset that I didn't stop by, and had blown the whistle. Bombshell of a letter I'd written. So much for trusting my intuition. My resource teacher at that school was called into the grizzly meeting, and rubbed it in after Mr. G had finished shredding me to pieces. She coldly informed me that the head of the project would be notified. Mr. G then added the frosting.

Kathy, you must never see that student again, or talk to his mother. For that matter, all of your counseling is suspended—indefinitely! In case the school is sued because of this letter, you will find no support here. Finally—and you can quote me—I don't believe in all this psychology, anyway! You may have a lot of booklearning, but you haven't lived. You're overzealous. Your heart may be in the right place, but not your judgment. Now, get out of here!

Numbly obedient, I turned to go sit in my supervisor's classroom waiting for her lecture. The tiny, stubby chairs put me right where I belonged—next to the floor. She stood in the darkened doorway a moment before strolling in to sit down on the table in front of me, not outwardly angry, but certainly not empathetic. I was very uncomfortable with her; she seemed to be gloating. She had nothing to say, and I silently stumbled out of the room in tears.

Before leaving the building, I went to my main supportive teacher's classroom, to tell her the news.

I got wind that something had happened involving Dwayne. The Big Man announced that none of the faculty was to be seen in company with you, Kathy. *Professionalism in education.*

The whole building is one mass of frustration anymore—I can hardly wait to get out of here! I'm just sorry this had to happen to you . . . *So was I. Glad it wasn't all my imagination!*

I resigned early the next week, leaving the circus a bitter eulogy:

To Whom It May Concern:

You win.

Any Other Song

>Because "my heart was in the
>right place, but
>not my judgment."

>You win.

>Because I was too dumb, too naive,
>too trusting, and
>"overzealous."

>You win.

>Because I tried too hard and
>lost the fight
>for body and mind.

>You win.

>But what about the kids?

    That horrible final week I'd been experiencing palpitations with my pulse zooming up to 160 and higher, which made me hyperventilate, my eyes blur, and nearly pass out. I kept attributing it all to a postencephalitic sequella—much more credible to me than anxiety. My distaste for food resulted in a weight loss of over 20 pounds, which I didn't mind. But the dullness drifted back to haunt me my last Friday at school. When I showed up for my part-time work at the hospital, Annie, gunner nurse and friend, saw that I wasn't quite myself. She did a dextro-stick and called Dr. Forster.
    He wasn't surprised to hear from us and was concerned that I wasn't doing too well. He referred me to an internist on call in the ER. That plan satisfied Annie, and she promptly escorted me downstairs. I'd been this route before . . .
    Kathy! What's going on? A short, mustached doctor was staring at my hyperventilating, withdrawn body, supine on the familiar stretcher in one of the same curtained-off cubicles of the Emergency Room. I'd had an EKG, been punctured for several tubes of blood, and jabbed with an IV.
    Hm? What's wrong with you? Why did you come to the Emergency Room? Why didn't you keep your appointment with Dr. Forster?
    I was sure glad my old neurologist had given this new doc my pertinent history so he'd be up on my case. He probably thought it was all in my head, too. He was grilling me about "what's wrong?" If I knew, I wouldn't be here. *I don't know.*

Look at me! You're hyperventilating. Just try and talk to me. Ok? *Dr. Reilley was insistent on not letting me just fade like I had before, as though it wasn't all something I had no control over.* Why did you call Dr. Forster today? *I was just so tired and cloudy inside.*

Don't you think that if someone of your intelligence presented to you in this manner, that you would be very concerned?

He wasn't going to let me vegetate at all. Things just went dizzy and blurry today. It was like trying to see through rippling water or something. A nurse I work with was concerned enough to call Dr. Forster, who referred me to you. So here I am. *I was afraid that if I told him I hadn't eaten all day or that nothing was going well anywhere, that he'd be convinced I was making myself sick and wouldn't look for another explanation. I sincerely wanted him to come up with a real cause for my recurrent spells.*

Your husband's a medical student. How're things going there? *Hey, world! Did you know I'm married to a med student? Dr. Reilley kept standing by the stretcher, waiting for me to open up. Something had to give, and it was me. I started crying. I didn't want to trust him, knowing he'd probably jump to all kinds of conclusions when I told him about* Ted's constant studying and preoccupation with perfection, and how he didn't come to see me enough while I was hospitalized, and rarely seemed to perceive, let alone talk to me. *And I suppose I wasn't trusting the situation at all to the Lord, either—He didn't seem to even be around since so many things had turned sour.*

You seem to be calming down now. Kathy, do you want me to be your doctor? *I nodded hesitantly—since when did they ask?* Then, if I'm going to treat you, you're going to have to agree to meet with a psychiatrist as well, or I won't continue to see you. Alright? *Shit!*

Tears welled up again inside as I realized I had no choice. I again nodded consent, breaking into sobs. To acknowledge that I needed psychiatric care was the hardest admission I ever made. It was one thing to accept the fact that some of my friends had seen a shrink, and understand that many people were helped by that kind of counseling. I wouldn't have studied psychology in college if I hadn't believed that it helped. But not me. Never me! How could God be asking me to undergo therapy? I could accept all of the times that I'd been injured and suffered disappointments because of my many accidents. I'd been able to endure that kind of pain. But what did He want with my mind? *How could crazy people be any kind of testimony to Him? I just couldn't do that. I was "the rock" . . .*

Any Other Song

> Consult note: 23-year-old female, wife of a medical student, referred to me by Dr. Forster (neurology). Patient presented 2 months ago with signs suggesting cerebellar tremor (abnormal discs, ataxia, headaches), was worked up in hospital with lumbar puncture, angiogram, etc., all normal. Hyperventilation occurred night before discharge, well documented. Since discharge, has not done well. Presented to ER with monocular blindness, felt hysterical by neurology (can't find chart—hearsay). Saw Dr. Forster one time after discharge. He presented idea may be a psychosomatic component. She rejected idea. Re-appointed after blindness episode to Dr. Forster. She didn't keep appointment. Left a letter saying if hysterical, will resolve. Valium prescribed for hyperventilation—made her high "like amphetamine." Over the past week increased frequency of episodes of hyperventilation. Talked with husband—he has documented sudden onset of heart rate at 160 and regular, associated with feeling of lightheadedness and lasting 5–10 minutes. Today, sudden onset while working, staff noted pulse at 120, increased rate regular, pale color, dextrostick 45%. Respirations 32 and shallow, 2+ carpal spasms, fundi with blurred discs, P 126, BP 124/92. Seemed withdrawn. Pushed glucose. ECG—tachycardia. Had long conversation with patient, symptoms gradually subsided. Impression: bizarre course of events over past month. Neuro findings unclear etiology. Rapid heart action sounds good for supraventricular tachycardia. Hyperventilation seems like acute anxiety attacks. Discussed anxiety with patient, willing to see Dr. Westberg for consultation. Will see in 2 weeks after complete lab workup.

Saturday morning I had the women in the Bible study group over for lunch, and was ecstatic BJ had consented to come. Everything seemed back to normal, casually conversing over ham and scrambled eggs. Jo, who hadn't been able to come, called a little later, while everyone was still there, and asked to speak with Lindy. It seemed innocent enough. They talked awhile, then Lindy said Jo wanted to talk to me, and she went upstairs to find Ted. That seemed strange.

What's going on, Jo?

Well, you know I'm on neurology this month, and BJ and I have both talked with the chief resident. Tears began to spill out as I sensed what was coming next. *Kathy, I really love you, but I just feel that you need to talk to a psychiatrist. Sometimes the Lord asks us to work things through with other people. And so on.*

That was when I seriously began to doubt if I had ever known me, after all. Was I really denying so many things? Why was the problem so blatantly obvious to everyone but me? It was embarrassing to be so upset in front of everyone, mostly because I prided myself on being one of the strong Christians in the group, always having an answer. But if everyone I respected thought I needed to see a shrink, then I'd have to go, because no one was going to come to me anymore for counseling or ask me for help in anything ever again. Always before I could be leaned on, trusted, and helpful to so many of my friends. What had happened? Was I making myself believe it was all organic and really suppressing something incredibly big? What? Lindy had confided to Ted that according to Jo, the docs had written it off as an hysterical conversion reaction. Was that really me? Those-in-white impressed upon Jo that they wanted to control it before it became a psychosis. I just felt lost.

BJ, why me? Why is God letting this happen to *me?* I desperately needed to know that someone there cared about me and understood my anxiety. But I was afraid to lean too heavily on BJ or Jo for fear of driving them away. No one had any answers, though . . .

Saturday's revelation faded and I felt like going out and getting roaring drunk that night. I just couldn't understand how or why the Lord would be allowing all of this to happen. It was as though I was expected to be someone or do something I knew I couldn't but should, and yet not really caring any more. Why couldn't He just leave me alone?

Monday I endured thyroid tests, the glucose-tolerance test, and whatever else Dr. Reilley had ordered, but I knew they would be negative, too, simply because everything else had been. I knew that's how God would work it out, and it made me angry. With much support from BJ, I resigned myself to seeing the psychiatrist, because those-in-white left me no alternative. My mind told me how miserably I'd failed to be to Ted all that he wanted and expected, which was why he wasn't enjoying my company any more. But I didn't care; I was tired of trying.

That whole week I dreaded going to see Dr. Westberg, and wanted badly for something to show up on the tests—anything subtle and serious. I told God I could accept that, but would never accept the possibility that my feelings were precipitating my symptoms. At our Bible study, I apologized for my past outbursts and tried to explain to each of them how awful things had been lately—having to resign at school, agreeing to see a shrink, feeling frustrated at my indifference to what I thought I should be and feel as a Christian. I couldn't tell what was going on in the minds of those medical students, though. BJ was there, silent, seeming to understand; but by the end of the week she'd be gone—moving out of state. It appeared that God was telling me I had no business depending on anyone—that He was sufficient. Right. But He

Any Other Song

wasn't tangibly there, and I needed somebody real to help. BJ was leaving, and I was scared.

The month finally ended the Monday after all of my lab tests, and I still didn't know why I was sick. As an appropriate gesture for starting out the new month, Ted and I kept the appointment with Dr. Westberg. Out of a vague curiosity, after reading all of my psychology texts, I'd always wanted to see what it would be like to be a patient seeing a psychiatrist—wondered how I'd respond. I just never thought I would really find out.

Since I hadn't started back full time at work, I'd been somewhere else. Ted was waiting for me, chatting with the doc as I blazed in out of the rain, panting and dripping. Wonderful first impression, but I like not to be forgotten. His office was in a second-floor wing of the old psychiatric hospital, up a crazy flight of chain-link-enclosed stairs. The walls were brown under a twelve-foot ceiling. Cheap chrome and plastic laminated furniture was sparsely arranged around a huge red-orange shag rug, which barely covered a black tile floor. There must have been fifteen feet between his chair and ours; distance obviously made him more comfortable. Westberg just sat over there—free-styled hair, corduroy sportcoat, cigarette smoke circling his tanned face. He seemed very young to be in his position as Director of Emergency Psychiatry.

Well. Why are you here?

I laughed at that stupid opener, and considered turning around immediately and leaving but changed my mind and plopped down in a chair to catch my breath and gather what intelligible thoughts I could.

Well. You can be damned sure it wasn't my idea! The docs said that unless I came to see you, they wouldn't treat me. So—here I sit. *I was going to have to be careful about what I said since shrinks have different tricks than the psychologists for squeezing out unconscious motives. Maybe Ted knew what they were, and that explained his silence. Except I was the patient—not him, unfortunately.*

All right, Kathy. I've looked over your chart, and I think your problem is indeed organic. I don't think you're a fake. Ok? *My defenses shot higher than ever, suspicious of his intentions.* First, I'd like to run through some problems with you. I'd like you to count backwards from 100 by 7s. *This was asinine!* Come on—100, 93 . . . Ok, Ok—so I'll count for you.

Fine. That's far enough. Next, I'd like you to interpret some parables for me. "A stitch in time saves nine." *Mom, you should be here for this—these games you'd really enjoy!* "You can lead a horse to water, but you can't make him drink." *You can make me come to see you, but you can't make me talk.* "People in glass houses shouldn't throw stones." *Just because you're clear-headed doesn't give you the right to expect more of me than is fair.*

After the amusing mental gymnastics, he stopped talking. *I wondered if that was my clue to start running off at the mouth, but I refused to verbalize with this stranger.*

Ted, would you mind stepping outside for awhile? *Ted shot him a dirty look as he left. Way to go!* Now then, Kathy. What haven't you told me?

I glanced unbelievingly around the room, thinking I must have misunderstood him. But he was intently serious. I stared at the rain-drenched trees outside the smudgy windows; they were barely budding in the afternoon spring. Just what is that supposed to mean?

In other words, are you having an affair, or have you had one in the recent past?*He nonchalantly turned on the fan in the smoky haze.*

An affair? Are you kidding? And neither have Ted and I ever considered divorce, like Dr. Forster implied. We don't happen to believe in such so-called alternatives. *What's with these people?*

I see. You think marriage is a sacred institution.*I nodded dumbly. I didn't see how in the world God would want us seeing this guy.* What's that fish you're wearing?

This answer was going to make me sound even crazier in the eyes of the medical profession. Christians, I thought, aren't supposed to ever be crazy enough to see psychiatrists. It's the symbol of early fundamental Christianity.

So, do you believe in the devil?

Well, of course! Don't you? You're Jewish, aren't you? *That set him back, but he waited for me to continue.* You see, I tried to explain to Dr. Forster all about what I thought had happened when I was hospitalized, but he just couldn't understand. Most docs probably don't believe in anything supernatural. Since there didn't seem to be an organic cause for my symptoms, I just assumed I had suffered a Satanic attack—it felt like something was trying to kill me when I had that respiratory arrest. I know that probably sounds strange to you, but that's the only explanation I have. *There! I'd said it all. He was pensive, but not apparently surprised. I didn't know what to think in the uncomfortable silence.*

That's quite interesting. You believe you're sick because of some transgression?

No! Just attacked because—well, because of who I might become.

Any Other Song

I see. Well, our time is up . . . I'd like to set you up for a battery of psychological tests so that we can better understand the problem. Ok? If there is anything organically wrong, these tests will find it. *That was smooth closure.*

What do they cover?

Generally, everything—personality, motor dysfunction, memory. *He was thumbing through his little brown book.* The earliest we can set it up is in four weeks. Would you and your husband be able to see me in two weeks, and then after your tests, we'll decide where to go from there. Ok? *Sure. Why not?* See you then.

Hadn't that been enlightening? Ted and I left in a mild state of shock. We should do this more often. It's easy to see how shrinks help so many people. And hanging in limbo—that was the best part.

SIX

a dandelion—weed
you say? but
the little girl's beaming
at her flower
fuzzy gold in the sun.
and a crabapple—not ripe
you say? but
see how she awes
at the color—Snow White reborn!
and the acorn—nothing
you say? yet
look at her eyes sparkle
with the magical find—a seed to plant,
an oak to grow.
then the feather—trash
you said, throwing them all away,
smashing her worthless dreams,
careless of her fantasy
while she gazed
in tears
as the duck down floated
to a gentler, warmer
hand.

One afternoon before BJ left, I ushered up sufficient courage to share with her my aching self-doubts, exposed since everyone had

Any Other Song

agreed I needed to see a psychiatrist. Perhaps, though, working on the neuro ward gave her a different perspective, or learned silence, because she said little about my emotional devastation—or hysteria. My verbiage must have confirmed her suspicions. Maybe she was just relieved to be going . . .

Watching. Everyone watching. That's how I felt when Ted and I doubled with Jo and Ron one night. They all reprimanded me for my inability to be what everyone expected me to be—a Christian. So I had a rotten time, and thought I might just leave them all as they sat munching in MacDonald's. Take off down the street, never to be heard from again. I wondered where the old, calm, coherent me had gone, or if that had merely been a façade. Maybe, when I didn't have the scrub oak bluffs to run to anymore, I started turning all that energy inside somewhere; and when I got the flu, it was an excuse to uncork the last several years of pent-up frustration and seething anger. Could that be why I wasn't well? Could I be that neurotic? I wasn't looking forward to seeing Dr. Reilley again to find out, either.

> Clinic visit: patient returns seemingly much improved. Lab tests done; one visit with Dr. Westberg past Monday. No more episodes of rapid heart action or hyperventilation, but has had episodes of more mild anxiety which are short lasting. Headaches also decreasing. Much warmer person today—smiling, talking freely, and feels that whole syndrome is getting better. She looks well, P 72, discs still blurred, Amphetamine screen negative. I absolutely do not know what's happened to this girl. A post-viral encephalitis syndrome is possible. Her personality is disturbing and I feel there is a good chance of deep-seated psychopathology, but I'm not at all convinced it is part of her recent maladies. Will see her again in two weeks for followup, but can see no other workup to proceed with now. Dr. Westberg will see her again.

I was feeling self-destructive on the way home from work the day I saw Dr. Reilley. Ted thought I'd been getting better, but I felt like it was all getting worse. Sometimes I wondered how together I was when for an afternoon I could be so high, when I was so down that same morning. And the very next day, when I thought it had all been cleared up, it would happen again. I wondered if I'd know whether I was crazy, or if it would just become impossible to keep things controlled—so those-in-white would be forced to put me away for awhile. Some days, things would just happen, and I didn't realize they were crazy until afterward. I almost wished that, for a little while, I would lose touch completely so that things wouldn't hurt so deeply. I was frustrated that I wasn't living as I knew I should be, but Ted didn't seem to even care. He was totally involved in his role as The Medical Student, and apparently felt I could handle it all. I always had. There didn't seem to be anyone I could talk to about how I was feeling. No one seemed to have any time for me. It was strange how, when I'd say some things it seemed so clear and real to me, yet no one else appeared to understand or even to have heard me. As long as everyone else was denying that something was wrong, it became hard to continue to think there was a reason to keep seeing my doc.

> Such a deal. Such a deal.
> Two-in-one. Such a
> deal.
> Once together, now another.
> What's wrong? they wonder
> Two-in-one. Such a deal.
> Such
> a
> deal.

> Clinic visit: pleasant discussion, quite revealing. Still with occasional periods of anxiety, now related to times of stress, like waiting for me, driving to work. Symptoms are mild. Complained of feeling like two different people; sometimes feels disconnected and flat, noting forgetfulness, and seems to be much of the time "on the edge," getting angry easily. Expressed sexual frustration as well. Exam is unchanged. Discs are still blurred, no vessel changes. Will reschedule after psychological testing and visit with Dr. Westberg.

All of the things that I'd been saying didn't matter, now seemed important and insurmountable. Ted was trying to adjust to the new me, but wasn't doing very well. After our second unsatisfying visit with Westberg, Ted said to me as we trudged to the car in the rain that he thought he was going crazy.

Terrific! I'm fighting to keep some semblance of normalcy in my life, and you start acting as though you're falling apart! *I didn't even want to think about it. We'd had a decent marriage until those-in-white said we needed counseling. When we didn't talk on touchy matters, all went smoothly enough. It always had. Maybe it had become just a game—living together, I mean. I blamed it all on medicine. As we drove, my mind wandered from the road off into a passing field where the grass had grown to a deep, lush green, the trees to a pale early summer lime.*

Any Other Song

When I showed up at 8 AM at the psych hospital for the marathon mental agility tests, I was a wreck. Outside it was cold and gray. The woman who was supposed to administer the battery was a few years older, which made me uneasy. I wanted to relate to her as a person to chat about the weather, compare jobs, be casual, but she wasn't comfortable with that.

She began by recording my complete social and medical history. She seemed incredulous at not having enough lines to write it all down.

I'm, uh, accident prone.

So I see. *She sat across from me behind a large wooden desk. The room was narrow, with the familiar twelve-foot ceiling.*

We whipped through over half of the tests by lunchtime; she gave me the personality inventory to keep myself occupied until we began again at 1:00. I wandered around the medical center and noticed that it had started raining. As the clouds turned blacker, hail erupted, pelting the lingering spring flowers. I went back early to finish the questionnaire, and by 3:00 I'd been tested for everything anyone could possibly imagine—from IQ to finger dexterity. At least it was over. Or have I said that before?

> Test results: this 23-year-old female earned verbal and performance IQ values which are both in the superior range, and the overall pattern yields no evidence of cerebral dysfunction. She did quite well on our detailed battery of neuropsychological tests—even for someone with her educational background. Therefore, it is our conclusion that she does not have a clinically significant cerebral lesion at this time. The personality profile, however, is usually seen associated with so-called "hysterical psychoses," or other borderline states. While not blatantly psychotic, such patients often experience "funny spells" involving dissociation, fugues, etc. which may provide mechanisms for withdrawing from unmanageable situations in their everyday lives. Frequently such patients come in with very unusual "neurological" symptoms, but these symptoms generally do not have an organic basis. There is likely to be a tremendous amount of denial around sexuality and aggression, and the patient appears to be under some pressure from basically unacceptable hostile impulses at this time. Religiosity is often seen with such patients—this may serve to impose some structure on their otherwise uncertain if not confusing views of life, and also fits in with the general tendency to deny or dissociate unpleasantness. The prospects for such patients making significant changes with therapy are usually not very good. Although they may become transiently psychotic at times, they generally pull together rather quickly, and their multiplicity of defenses allows them to persist at that level. In addition, they tend to resist psychiatric treatment.

E. J. Daniel

Ted and I went together again to see Westberg a week after my tests, and he assured me that all the tests were negative. I was thrilled.

Feel free to come in and see me again, but when you do, *both* of you have to come. Otherwise, there's no reason to continue our sessions since the test results were not indicative of any organic etiology.

Well, I don't believe, Dr. Westberg, that there was a reason to come see you in the first place. I just do not believe in psychotherapy. *Ted sure told him. Guess we weren't ever coming back, then.*

On a too-hot cloudless day I returned to see Dr. Reilley. He seemed very intent, almost studying me before finally deciding to do a superficial exam. He was certainly taking his time.

Kathy, I want you to know that I really enjoy seeing you, and do come in and see me whenever you want to. But medically, I can't justify asking you to return for follow-up.

There you have it—the end of all my visits with all my doctors.

> Clinic visit: fundi unchanged. Much more open. Psych evaluation complete; she is disappointed not to be able to see Dr. Westberg again. Has tenderness left posterior neck—think muscular. Recommend aspirin, heat and rest. Return prn.

As I studied myself in the mirror that night, it occurred to me that those-in-white weren't telling me the truth. I was really experiencing a sort of general body failure. They were playing out their parts as God, and I was the pawn. I realized there were times when I wasn't aware of things, but I had no idea how serious it had gotten until I tried to remember what I'd done or where I'd been. I imagined myself as having a serious and undetectable lesion somewhere—and no one could find it. They had all given up. And Ted said he loved me too much—that's what was wrong between us. But I knew better.

It was all quite confusing. It appeared that sanity (or insanity) was based largely on someone else's perception; that my most intimate, introspective thoughts and feelings were no longer in my jurisdiction; and that the verdict—sane or insane—was not my decision, but would be handed down from those-in-white. In fact, I was not even being consulted. I didn't know how it would all eventually work out, and the loneliness and isolation deepened.

> would that i was someplace else
> where i once was

Any Other Song

*and no one else could
know or hurt
the part of me
that mattered most.*

*once
i was alive
but that was taken
away
leaving me with only
skeletons and
nothing to build
tomorrows.*

*and it came to pass
that in the latter days
my inside
self-destructed
and i never knew
the other side
that managed
to survive.*

SEVEN

After the ego-shattering ordeal, I just needed to get away from it all and think, so I vacated to the northwest coast. The ocean had always been soothing to me, and I desperately wanted to feel the deep damp mist brought inland by brisk morning breezes, my body perched on some beached driftwood, inhaling the salt-fish air, exhilarated by the expanse. Actually, it was a good excuse to see my folks.

My visit was complicated when, skipping along a patch of windworn rocks and scotchbroom, I tripped and fractured my foot. My parents were concerned, but hardly surprised. Neither was I. I guess God wasn't finished with me yet.

Mom said it wouldn't have been a typical visit if I hadn't hurt myself. At least my orthopedic doc, once I returned home, was unaware of my previous mental duress, and treated me as a normal casualty. The accident seemed justification enough to Ted that I shouldn't have gone without him, because my injuries always seemed to happen when he wasn't there. He wanted to protect me, he said, but that didn't make sense to me since he hadn't really been around to do anything since he'd been in med school.

While on the coast, I didn't spend as much time as I should have sorting out my feelings. Running was preferable, and trying to accept that I might be having marital problems was just a deterrent.

Any Other Song

From every objective point of view, Ted was part of the reason I was sick. But that ran contrary to everything I knew as a Christian. But then, maybe I didn't know, anymore. In fact, I didn't really know anything anymore. I just knew that I'd started drinking heavily, for whatever reason. That wasn't wise, but I couldn't find another way to cope, and knowing that it made Ted furious gave me a strange sense of satisfaction. I knew, too, it had been a long time since I'd felt caged—since high school, maybe. My impatience between finishing one thing and getting on with the next—out of high school, out of college, into marriage—amazed my Mom. Maybe I'd been repressing so many feelings that I'd become saturated to the point of exploding. But I didn't understand how I couldn't be conscious of what was going on inside. How could I not know when I was suppressing something, and when I wasn't? Certainly I was more attuned to myself than that. Or was that a delusion? People at work suggested giving Ted an ultimatum—either shape up or I split. But they didn't believe he would ever change. After all, hadn't I done everything I possibly could? I'd submitted, for awhile; I'd taken classes to learn to be what he wanted me to be, and put those principles into practice, for awhile; I'd talked to counselors about what to do; I'd even waited, for awhile. When none of those things worked, I thought I might just leave without giving him a choice. Maybe that would turn him around. I believed he had the problem. I thought he was an emotional wreck. And I continued to drink, especially the nights he was on call.

Several weeks after my summer excursion, our problems as a couple seemed to intensify. I had thought that by getting away for a few days things would cool down, or warm up—anything. I was upset that our once-deep relationship was gone—forever, it seemed. And I quickly learned the difference between helping someone and hurting them. Lindy wasn't the one to dump my garbage onto. That wasn't like me to be so insensitive, but the damage had already been done. Lindy told me she would never consider marriage now.

Because of the way I was portraying life at home, friends told me that Ted was more thin-skinned than they'd thought, and it would take a long time, if ever, for him to resolve his feelings of resentment and to satiate his craving for recognition. "Instead of leaving him, Kathy, be more gentle, more flexible. Hang on a few more years until he finishes his training, and then everything will be alright." But they never said what I was supposed to do with myself in the interim.

Then one Thursday night when Ted was too tired, too distant, too whatever in response to my efforts at making up for nights past, I vowed that I'd get back at him for that. I'd make him sorry. His denial was confirmation enough that he was in love with medicine, and I no longer meant anything to him.

Friday evening, when Ted was again on call, I went out with my next door neighbor. It seemed deliciously secretive, in a way, and Steve and I had drinks before, during and after dinner. When we finally made it home, we topped it off by going skinny-dipping, and making love in the shimmering, silent moonlight. Assuring me he understood how lonely I'd been, he went home. When he'd gone, I cried bitterly, jolted into a realization that all of the problems I'd attributed to Ted were actually mine. It was a classic case of projection. I'd never thought twice about this one-night stand with Steve, nor the consequences of my vengeance. I'd been able to detach myself from the part of me that could have stopped it all before it was too late. I'd willfully chosen to do what I believed was terribly wrong, and hadn't cared! Everything I had ever valued I'd just destroyed, and I waited for God to destroy me. I prayed and prayed for forgiveness, knowing that I couldn't forgive myself, afraid I wasn't sorry.

The next week I daily tried to resolve my deepening guilt, knowing in my head that it was theoretically forgiven, but that didn't make it real for me. The world would say I was justified, but that didn't erase my despair. Friends at work joked about how when I first started there I was a religious fanatic, but that thankfully, they had corrupted me, so now I fit in. The person I used to be had lost the battle.

Perhaps what I'd suppressed was now and forever who I would be. As I was tearfully contemplating that prospect, Nance, one of Jo's classmates and friends, asked me to lunch. When you start losing control of everything, with mere threads holding you together, you feel transparent enough so everyone sees the crack, too. It's so obvious when they're talking behind your back, shooting curious glances at you, not asking you anywhere anymore, generally pretending you're not even there. Then I wondered whether my imagination or my detachment made it seem that way. But I was still surprised I told Nance the story, as best I could, yet without the awful words the shrink used, or the labels Ted stuck on me. It was never an affair. I was not an alcoholic.

I think it's time to talk with Miriam, Kathy. Nance and I were sitting in the hospital cafeteria, and I was trying not to make a scene sobbing.

On Friday afternoon Jo drove me to meet Nance at Miriam's

Any Other Song

home. They hadn't given her the details, nor had I told Jo what exactly was wrong. I didn't have to. I just pleaded with her to not be angry with me when it was all said. It had become impossible for me to look anyone in the face.

Kathy. I want you to tell me everything, every part of it. Now is not the time to be reserved and withdrawn. We want to help. *Miriam's blunt seriousness was terrifying. As I tried to relate what I'd done, I began to cry. I wanted my vulnerability to be obvious, so they wouldn't hurt me more than I was already hurting. I wanted so badly to get up from the carpeted, sun-filled den where the four of us sat around the table, wanted to excuse myself, to burst out of the warmth and run, run, run. I never wanted to see those knowing, loving faces again, yet my mind knew that I had to face what had happened. But it was all too terrible. To soften the blows I thought were coming my mind drifted off, and I was unable to hear all that was said to me. By telling them, though, it had become less a game, less something it was possible to hide.*

Maybe it would help if you got away, just to think about what you want to do, Kathy. *Miriam looked intently at me. She knew! She'd been there, too, in a way, and I could feel her reaching inside, touching my terror and pain. But I could never tell Ted, which she said would be necessary. Nor would I be able to find the strength or resolve to tell Steve I could never see him again. Out of deep concern, she was relentless.*

I walked away more numb than when I'd arrived, unable to reply to Jo. Oh, Kathy! When and where is this going to stop?

By Sunday I knew I was losing. Ted was on call again, and in an attempt to find new strength, I drove our truck to the mountains, groping for answers. I hadn't planned very well where I was going, thinking it was a shorter distance than it turned out to be. I stopped several times along the dirt road of the timberline pass to let my dogs run, taking occasional pictures as though it was a trip to be remembered. But there were too many other people, so I pulled off onto a barely visible jeep track etching up the mountainside between stands of white barked, golden-green aspen. I crawled out of the cab and sat down on a tree trunk to wait for an inspiration or a revelation, or maybe, finally, peace. A piercing ringing in my ears persisted, and I could only cringe in a vague uneasiness. This made the trip anything but an escape and a chance to sort out the confusion.

After many restless minutes, I jumped back in the truck. Getting off the mountain became a nightmare—every turn I rounded on

E. J. Daniel

the narrow rutted road offered a grotesque temptation to drive off and over the treeless cliff, tumbling into painless oblivion. If I'd had more courage, or hated myself more, or wanted to spite those who'd said I'd get through it all right in the end, maybe I would have heeded the nagging urge to crash and burn.

Much later I finally got home, and badly needed calming. I took up my familiar habit; there hadn't been a day in the last two months that I hadn't had at least two drinks, usually more. I didn't have a craving for it, just a reverence for the state of euphoria it brought, no matter that it was only transient. It was better than nothing.

Maybe it was just the suggestion that the doctors had made, or maybe it was there all along, but I was ready. Ted hardly seemed to notice my growing disillusionment. He'd forsaken me for his medical career, forcing me to look elsewhere for some meaning to my life, and by then I was desperate. Perhaps the irony was the distant warning from Miriam spoken so early in the summer: "Whatever you do, Kathy, don't invite him inside your home." Was it worth the price?

and the lack of His discipline
is excrutiating
not even recognizing
the symptoms of grave
error, so i ran
desperately groping
for any peace
but finding only more
uncertainty.

the gulf i created
between myself and too many others
because of that error hurts
endlessly;

but i'm scared and so
ashamed,
and don't know how
to bridge the
chasm
between where i should be
and where i am.

someone, please, help
me, tell me
how to make the tears and

Any Other Song

> *eonic pain*
> *disappear, and heal*
> *the wounds*
> *that now scar*
> *those i thought*
> *i loved.*

I'd been avoiding Steve all weekend but he knew Ted's schedule, so he dropped by our apartment in the middle of my Sunday drunk. I told him that it was all a mistake, that I was sorry I caused him any grief, and to go away and leave me alone. I even closed the door on him as he was asking if we couldn't still be friends. Turning around from the door, there seemed to be only one answer.

Dumb for me, maybe, because I was "too intelligent"—but dumb was all I was now. I popped all of the pills in our medicine cabinet. I was unhappy and miserable, and I knew I could never, never confess to Ted what I'd done. I'd failed him, failed my friends, failed myself. I wished I'd died six months earlier in the hospital. At least it would have saved me and everyone else from all the hell I'd created. I thought of all the people I'd known that had committed suicide, and finally understood how they'd gotten to that point.

When I'd drunk enough with the pills to start feeling really sick, I quit—partly in fear—realizing what I was trying to do. I stumbled upstairs to lie down and tried to call Nance, but she wasn't home. Ted called me a little later, but he couldn't tell that anything was wrong and wasn't coming home as I'd planned, so I didn't tell him. I just hung up, in tears, and prayed that God wouldn't let me die. But if I did, that was alright because I certainly deserved it.

> Crumpled under the towering fir, she sobbed into the cushiony pine needles. She had felt it would happen before it actually did and it might have been her loneliness or curiosity that had gotten the better of her rational self. And that ghost would haunt her forever. Through the falling mist she remembered waiting for her parents in the musty church parlor during their weekly evening choir rehearsals. She missed that warm time long past. As she lay on the antique couch, the counterpoint of a distant fugue lingered in her mind. . . .

> *warm*
> *blows the wind*

E. J. Daniel

in a summer dream
tossing wisps
through powder sky
playing wistfully
in mind and matter.

soft
melts a sunset
orange into dusk
after tormenting showers
raged into pain
offering solace
to a crying
child.

CONSIDER

1. Try to pinpoint the stressors that triggered Kathy's paranoia and developing pathological depression. What crises can be identified as situational? As developmental?
2. Harrison* includes the following residual symptoms of encephalitis: "mental deterioration, amnesiac defects, personality change, and hemiparesis. There is wide variation in the incidence of latent changes depending on the type of viral infection." How could a differential diagnosis of encephalitic sequellae vs. a manipulative behavior be supported?

---

*Ibid.

EIGHT

The faded orange light of dawn woke me up, alone and intensely hung over. I'd tried to plan last night's disaster so that Ted would come home and find me. That would have been my way of telling him that everything was not alright, contrary to his belief. But God didn't let it turn out that way. I'd expected to wake up in the hospital where those-in-white would keep me from doing to myself what I'd tried to do Sunday. I wondered if anyone really cared. But no one knew. They probably all figured that it could happen to other people, but not to Kathy. She was too smart to do a crazy thing like that. She's not suicidal. Maybe if someone needed me desperately enough, I'd break out of my woe-is-me syndrome, but it seemed to be my turn to play the despairing role. I suppose it could have been a game I played—a part of me that didn't know how deadly it could be. I was thankful, in a way, that God let me wake up. But having no one there made me feel more isolated than last night.

After trying to sober up, I tried calling Nance again, on the premise of inviting her over, earlier than arranged, for my holiday get-together.

Good morning, Nance! Did I get you up?

No, but you sure sound tired.

Yeah, in a way. I tried calling you last night, but you weren't there. *I was angry.*

Any Other Song

Kathy. What are you trying to say?

Oh, I, uh, got very depressed yesterday after taking a drive in the mountains, and I started drinking last night when I got back because I was so uptight. Then Steve came by, like you all knew he would, and I tried—I really tried to tell him everything the way Miriam told me to, and he said he still wanted to be friends. I even shut the door on him, and it was too much that I didn't need, and—I took a bunch of pills.

There was a long silence. Why, Kathy? Did you have a headache?

No, Nance. You know what was happening.

No, I don't. You tell me. What were you trying to do?

Now that I had her on the phone, it was a lot harder to actually put into words what I'd tried to do. I felt bad for even calling her, half ashamed, half afraid. I guess I wanted to die. No one was home. Ted called and said he had to stay at the hospital after all, and no one was here to help. So why should I even care? Things just aren't working out Nance!

I think what you're going through is that emotional storm Miriam warned you about.

I didn't even hear that part.

There were a lot of things you probably didn't hear. Maybe you could call her and talk to her about what's going on right now.

Oh, I don't know . . . I don't feel too hot. Besides, I don't want to bother her on a holiday. I'll just see you later on.

You'll be alright?

Sure . . .

I was too sick to attempt anything more. Anyway, I felt compelled to make a valiant try at having everything ready in time for the barbeque. Ted sauntered in around 10:30 that morning, and hit the bed. He didn't even notice that I wasn't myself. Fine. I was a better actress than I thought, but I still resented him for not seeing. After Nance and Lindy arrived, I busied myself in the kitchen, avoiding Nance. Ted finally roused himself in time to visit with Jo and Ron, and that added diversion helped. No one else apparently had been clued in, and Nance and I continued to pretend everything was just fine. Midway through the afternoon, I was propped up against the kitchen wall trying to regain my stamina when Lindy poked her head around the corner.

Kathy! Are you feeling alright?

No, but I'll tell you about it later. Thanks, anyway.

They all seemed to have had an enjoyable time, in spite of the fact they were in the midst of finals. That was another reason I found not to tell Ted, because I knew he wouldn't be able to take the rest of his exams if he knew about Steve or Sunday—or anything.

Tuesday I went to work, afraid to stay home even though I still felt heavily drugged. One of our doctors approached me to ask some piddling question, and I found myself backing away from him. He just stared at me like I was crazy.

What in the world is wrong with you, Kathy?

I just don't feel too good. *I thought I was going to explode.*

Well, I'm having trouble finding that letter you typed for me. Come over to my office and show me where you put it.

It's right on top of your desk!

I can't find it. Will you please come show me where it is?

I stormed over to his office, irate that he could be so blind. When he shut the door behind us, I realized he was only trying in an inconspicuous manner to get me out of the lab, so we could talk.

Now, what is going on? I've never seen you like this! *He motioned me to sit down, genuinely concerned. I couldn't even get out two sentences before I broke into embarrassing sobs. Not as tough as I thought, no longer a rock, no more knowing what to do. I told him about Sunday.*

Oh, my God! If I were Ted, I'd sure as hell want to know about that. If he doesn't think you're more important than his career, and I'm not belittling him, then he doesn't deserve to be married to you. He's going to have to figure out his priorities. Jesus, Kathy!

That's quite right. But it doesn't help me. *I couldn't tell Ted. Miriam said that when I did get around to telling him, it shouldn't be in anger, but out of forgiveness, and deep remorse. That would hurt.*

Wednesday night I happened to see Ted outside, walking the dogs, talking with Steve. I almost screamed, but they acted as though there was nothing wrong, as if nothing had ever happened. I finished the drink I was holding, fixed another, inhaled it, and sloshed together another, popping some aspirin to fend off a headache. I had eased into the couch when Ted came in.

What are you doing?

Sulking.

What's wrong with you?! *That meant: I am concerned but not enough to hang around for your answer.*

If I tell you, will you promise to listen and not get all upset?

Well, of course. You can tell me.

That probably wasn't a fair or reasonable request, since he was already irritated that I was drinking, but my defenses were down

Any Other Song

enough, my restraints shot, to not care about what I was saying. I started with Sunday night, and before he could recover from that shock, I told him what had prompted it. I'd gotten and kept his attention alright. He'd been ignoring me all summer, so I went out on him, and when that didn't do the trick, I kept on. But it backfired. I had his attention for all the wrong reasons. When I'd tried to be what God wanted me to be, Ted took me for granted, expecting even more of me. That left me the alternative of being someone else who could restore some meaning to the marriage.

I'm not taking my final tomorrow. I can't . . . And I'll just take the next two weeks off and spend the time with you. Ok?

That'll mess up your whole schedule!

Kathy! I want to help. It's probably all my fault it happened, anyway. *He succeeded in making me feel sorry for him, regretful that I'd hurt him. I really did want him to do* something, *though, to help me, to help us. We used to be so close, and could tell each other anything, and solve all the problems. How had we lost it?*

The next morning he called our pastor, but I never heard the results of their conversation. No counseling was ever arranged. I told Miriam that I'd finally confessed to Ted, and she suggested that we both come over to talk things out, which Ted reluctantly agreed to do. I didn't understand why he was so hesitant to take any definitive action. He refused to say anything to her, leaving me to do all of the talking. He acted as though nothing was wrong with him, as though I was solely the one in dire need of counseling and he'd only brought me there to get well.

A week had passed since the revelation, and we took off for a short trip to try and paste the pieces together. When I packed the food box, I made sure I brought along my well-tried method of coping, dreading the time alone that we both would have to share. The radio filled in the long periods of driving in silence. When we'd stop to take pictures, he would urge me to come closer to the cliff edge and "look down there!" but I was terrified I would jump off. It wasn't until the fourth day, on our way home, that I was able to be cordial toward him, and it sort of made the entire camping trip worthwhile. Unfortunately, just when we might have been getting somewhere, he started back to class.

Thursday night I was alone again, Ted was on call, and maybe because I was angry or just wanted to run, I began mixing it up again. I wasn't trying to die, necessarily, but I didn't feel I could face things. I kept waiting for God to do something to me so I wouldn't hurt, but He just seemed so very far away. I ingested enough to grog myself into unconsciousness, scared and depressed.

Friday, my hangover and I went in to see Dr. Reilley again, because he'd said to come in whenever I needed to. Besides, I remembered he had said how much he enjoyed seeing me, and since Ted had failed to get me help, someone needed to keep me from destroying myself. I felt embarrassed having to tell the nurse that I just wanted to talk to him, and she left me to pace around the room.

Then he came in, a big grin blazing under his trimmed moustache. Hi, Kathy. Good to see you again! How are things?

I tried to return his smile, but could only look down at the floor. Well, I went to Walk-In Clinic a week and a half ago, and they said I had possible sinusitis or something, but the pills they gave me didn't work. So I thought I'd see you for follow-up.

And how's everything else? *He pulled the hair out of my face so he could see the tears I was trying to hide. I told him about the events of the past month. He didn't seem surprised.*

Would you mind if I had Dr. Westberg talk to you right now? Will you be alright sitting here, while I go call him, because I think you really need to see him.

I felt sick. I didn't think I was that *bad. As soon as he left to call my old shrink, I almost snuck out the back hallway, pretending I hadn't even bothered to come in. I paced furiously around the small, square examining room, looking at myself in the mirror, trying to see what had alarmed Dr. Reilley so. In the middle of one of my wild roamings he opened the door, expecting to see me sitting sedately in the chair where he'd left me. His sudden entry made me jump.*

Oh. There you are. Dr. Westberg is out of town, but one of the psych nurses is a good friend of mine, and she's willing to talk with you right now. Ok? She's over in the Emergency Room. *No! One of the docs at work was taking us out to lunch, and I knew if I could just get a couple of quick martinis down I'd be better.*

How about if I see her later this afternoon? I, uh, really need to get back to work.

You don't look in any state to work. I'll let you go only if you promise to come back down here at 2:00. If you don't show, I'll call you up and find out why. *I had no intention of talking to a strange nurse about my problems. Actually, I couldn't figure out why I'd gone down there in the first place. Things weren't that bad, really. What could I expect Dr. Reilley to say, anyway? I smiled meekly at him, and almost ran out of the clinic annex.*

Any Other Song

> Clinic visit: scheduled to see me this AM for follow-up from lymph swelling and nasal discharge not responding to ampicillin and actifed. Real reason to see me—very depressed. OD attempt Labor Day and attempted 2 times since. Doubt suicidal potential. Dr. Westberg is out of town—will ask our ER Psych service to see.

The martinis did help, and I suppose I was calling Dr. Reilley's bluff by not showing up as arranged. I just wanted to know how much he did care. He called.

Kathy, what happened to you?

I'm Ok now. *I didn't tell him why.*

Are you sure?

I'll be alright, really.

I want you to call me over the weekend, though, if you have any problems at all. I've arranged for Dr. Westberg to see you on Monday, and I've already contacted him about you.

That made me feel really stupid for having told him everything. I was deathly afraid of suicide, and at the same time I denied the possibility that it could be fatal. But by then, I'd almost forgotten the pain of my moonlit incident. Not knowing why, I continued to spend time with Steve, and Ted continued to spend time at the hospital. I thought about the impact it all had on Ted, and when I got home, helped myself to several more thought suppressants. When Ted arrived, he just ignored me, knowing that I would drink anyway in spite of all the Freudian crap he kept handing me (as though he was immune to any neuroses himself just because he was doing his rotation in Psychiatry).

You don't even know what you're doing to yourself! I can't believe you're turning into a real alcoholic! *His screaming accusation cut deep, but it hurt worse because I was powerless to stop myself.*

Because the pain of remembering things was becoming too much, I stopped remembering. Rehashing how I was feeling wasn't getting me anywhere, and by simply refusing to remember, it made the feelings less intense. On my way into the lab Monday morning, I whizzed by my old attending—Dr. Forster—who looked every bit like a frazzled nerve ending. I was shocked he recognized me, and even casually asked how I was doing. Just fine, thank you. He obviously didn't care, nor did anyone—at least not enough to help. Then Dr. Westberg called. "Hear you've been having some problems." No kidding. Where did you hear a crazy thing like that? He couldn't see me until Wednesday, again in the same bare-walled office. As proof of my short and bittersweet visit, he put me on anti-psychotic medication, and wanted both Ted and me there on Friday to see how we weren't operating as a couple. I felt big-time seeing a shrink twice that week, but more curious as to how the new pills and booze would mix.

Dr. Reilley was on vacation the following week, so I went back to Medical B with my chronic head symptoms. The nurse practitioner, after examining me, was gone a long time with my chart, though, and I began to get a little nervous. She finally returned, seeming oddly distant, followed by some doc.

We've just been reviewing your chart, and . . .

Great! And you think it's all in my head, too. Right?

Well, we're not sure, so we want you to be seen in the ENT clinic. By the way, why aren't you seeing Dr. Reilley?

He's on vacation.

They ordered another series of sinus films, which would naturally be negative. This was getting old, but I went to clinic the next day anyway, because I didn't want it said that I wasn't doing everything I could or was told to do to help myself. I even had the rare experience of being examined by a medical student, who unwittingly reviewed the psych test results with me, and other innocent data.

When I went back to see Dr. Westberg on Friday, I was prepared to elicit the truth about my prognosis. Those-in-white had lied to me.

In the first place, that medical student was out of line reading those interpretations to you. Second, I didn't ask for that particular test to be administered—it's just part of the battery, and not very reliable. I don't give the MMPI any credence. *He was avoiding the issue.*

After Dr. Reilley got back from his three-week vacation, I went to see him again. I much preferred his warm and comfortable approach to Westberg's iciness. Maybe he'd have some answers, or some direction that was lacking with the shrink.

Kathy, in a way I'm just barely able to cope myself. I don't have any answers for you. I wish I did. If I had a magic solution, I'd certainly share it with you. But I don't. All I can say is that if you attempt again, please come to my Emergency Room, so I can take care of you. *Thanks. If I have any choice in the matter, I'm sure I will.*

> Clinic visit: no exam today. Just talked about what's going on currently. Return prn.

Knowing where the only other answers might come from, I called Miriam. She offered to see me on Saturday.

Any Other Song

I got up early that morning to get all my piddly work done before I went over for the grilling. Miriam had all the directions, but I wasn't able to translate them into action. The hours passed quickly, part of me somewhere else, unable to remember much. I went home thoroughly convicted, but Miriam knew I wasn't convinced. It was disappointing, because I really wanted to feel better. She'd given me a plan: dump the liquor, pitch any reminders of the affair, completely cut off seeing Steve, and check in regularly with her. We wrote out my alternatives, but I was unable to assure her that suicide wasn't one of them.

Sunday I tried to keep busy in light of my new vows, but by 2:00 I'd run out of things to do, so I called Lindy. We talked for about half an hour, and she suggested that I do something physically active—after pouring out the alcohol. She sounded encouraged that I'd been able to do most everything else on Miriam's list. After hanging up, I obediently went into the kitchen, and literally turned my head as I emptied the bottles down the sink. All I could think of was how much money was pouring down the drain. Then I went outside for a bike ride in the warm, autumn sun. In the park I sat and meditated in the fallen cottonwood leaves, almost forgetting what was happening, watching the clouds make pattern after blurry pattern in the pale blue sky.

I went alone to see Dr. Westberg on Tuesday. I'd talked to him on the phone on Friday after Reilley had called him, concerned that I might OD that weekend. But when he prescribed more pills for me (which I didn't need but gladly accepted on the supposition I might leave town for awhile), I knew it was no big deal to him what happened. I hadn't told him I wasn't taking the pills regularly, and having even more at my disposal gave me a strange sense of security. We agreed that little progress was being made, and he suggested I just see Miriam for a month. In fact, it had already been arranged by phone, and they were in agreement I should see her instead.

Kathy, I have tried to get you to accept that a trial separation is better than suicide, but you reject that. I don't have any other answers for you. I think you value Miriam's opinion more than mine, so I'll just see you again one month from today. Since she can't prescribe more pills for you, call me when you need more. *I felt bad that he was giving up, even though we didn't seem to be getting anywhere. Sort of like when my orthodontist gave up after four years: "You just have a problem that can't be completely corrected." It's most encouraging.*

It made me a little uncomfortable that Miriam was already

aware of the arrangement, not knowing what kind of information the two professionals had shared. I told her I was going on a short trip with Nance and Lindy; she seemed relieved I was going away for a change of tempo, even if it was only four days. I felt like I needed weeks, maybe months. She wanted assurance from Nance and Lindy, though, that my going wouldn't worry them, or put a strain on our friendship. But they made me feel very wanted, and that was all I needed.

*At our Saturday marathon, Miriam had said "a person of your caliber, Kathy, just doesn't make such foolish decisions as you've been making." Everyone seemed to have such high expectations for me. I guess I wanted to rebel against the stereotyping, unhappy over not handling things in a manner becoming to a person with my supposed level of intelligence, drive and personality. But maybe I was simply unable to do all of the things everyone said would help get me out of my depression. I tried taking my coffee breaks and lunch hours privately, spending time reading scripture, fervently seeking any answers from the Lord. I even stood up in church Sunday night to testify that, "yes, it's been hard, but I'm on my way out of the pit"—no matter how tenuous that was. Inside I desperately wished that it **was** true, that I'd be alright, for everyone else's sake. Certainly not for mine, nor for Ted's necessarily, because I wasn't sure if I even loved him anymore, but I did care about Nance, Lindy and Miriam. I couldn't disappoint them; but I wasn't sure if I even had the energy to keep from failing the very people who wanted to help me the most. By going on that trip, I hoped to circumvent any irrational decisions. Maybe things would work out.*

We got a late start Thursday morning, but the long drive went quickly—too quickly, almost. The sky stayed a faded blue with wind-driven stringy clouds for miles and miles. Patches of stale, crusted snow still nestled in the deep arroyos along the highway, which stretched endlessly over the juniper mesa. I was surprised we found so much to talk about between all of our picture-taking stops. As the sky turned a brilliant yellow-orange as far as we could see, the eastern mountains pinked up from the sandia sunset, mellowing the vividness with its dusty cliffs. I should have melted into that quiet, dreamy twilight.

While they interviewed at the hospitals, all I could think about was the little girl I used to babysit for there, who'd died of leukemia, and Pattie, a family friend we'd grown up with, turned vegetable in a car accident recently. Her mom was empathetic to my depres-

sion, telling me how she had been suicidal trying to accept the fact that her 18-year-old daughter could never be rehabilitated. I felt guilty for having even considered dying, thinking about the anguish it might cause my mom. I determined to try even harder to beat that destructive part of me.

The trip turned out to be mildly cathartic, especially since it took us four hours longer coming home than going. It didn't bother any of us; it just happened. While we'd been enjoying the Indian summer, it had snowed in the mountains, and the pass glistened, incredibly silent. I wanted to stay there, at the summit, forever. Just to have everything stop. But I got too cold standing out in the frozen snow bank, and it really couldn't end there, anyway. So the three of us talked awhile before driving on in the eerie twilight.

Monday Ted decided it would be prudent if we moved closer to the medical school, so I began hunting for a new apartment. In the transition, I met again with Miriam. Nance had told her I'd been a "real blessing" on the trip, and that it wouldn't have been fun at all if I hadn't gone along. That warmed me inside, hearing that, but it didn't change the way things were at home. I confessed how I'd inadvertently accepted another date with Steve. She was incredulous.

Kathy! When are you going to stop complicating matters? Get out of that relationship before it's too late.

I'm afraid it already is.

What do you mean? *I suddenly felt very ill.*

It's been 7 weeks since I had my period. *Why am I still alive? I thought Miriam was going to start crying for me.*

Have you seen a doctor?

No.

Then I don't think it will help you right now if we keep on since we don't know for sure. Let's wait until we know, and go from there.

The following morning I cornered Dr. Reilley in the Emergency Room, and told him the news, trying to maintain my composure.

Is it Ted's? *Shit! When does it end?*

I don't know.

Well, there'll be no problem arranging for a therapeutic abortion with Dr. Westberg. Pregnancy's the last thing you need at this point. Wait another week, and then we'll check everything out. *Just like that.*

Friday I went to lunch with my sister and, naturally, had a drink. We met again after work for Friday Afternoon Club (happy hour) and I had at least five or six or more, mixing it up with my little blue pills that I always carried "for the panicky feeling." The more I *drank, the more I could admit what a rotten person I was, totally incapable of being what I knew I should be. Listening to the jazz pianist in the emerald green dullness of the bar made me feel that what I once had going for me was lost forever. I really missed that ability, that drive that could have made me, say, a decent musician who brought enjoyment to people instead of grief. And I drank more to avoid the pain of seeing what I wasn't. Talking about it made it worse; it was easier to deny that there was anything seriously amiss, easier not to face up to the failures. But inside, I knew I couldn't continue to avoid the facts, because somewhere something said it wasn't right. Where that voice came from, though, I never knew.*

At the apartment later that evening, Ted and I had a rerun of the boy-you-make-me-mad-when-you-drink script, and he almost took my pills, except that he felt I needed them. What a laugh. I didn't care about what he thought, anyhow, thinking I might just leave.

Then I began reasoning that the problem was that I wasn't disciplined. That was why I was having so much trouble not contemplating suicide as my way out. That was the easy solution. What I wanted was to succeed at something for a change—overdosing, but maybe be found in time and taken care of. Get help that seemed more real than what I'd been getting. I suppose I was wanting anyone to make me better, instead of me having to do it all by myself, because I didn't feel that I could. I wanted help. I needed it. I didn't feel I could change. I wanted to run, and drank instead; but somehow I couldn't just let go and do something crazy. My insides said I was more responsible than that. It was a horrendous battle, and I was so tired. I hated myself even more when I saw how depressed Nance had been lately. Not only did that hurt, because I couldn't help her when she needed it the most, but moreover because I'd contributed to her depression. I'd been leaning on her too heavily, assuming she could handle it. There are too many stumbling blocks already for me to hang around and be another.

nine

It was a cold, rational decision that I finally made. To die. Nothing mattered to me anymore and never would. No one was going to be able to help me or stop me; God had given up, so there was no reason to keep on trying.

Friday morning I returned to clinic to see Dr. Reilley, to tell him I wasn't pregnant after all—just an emotional wreck. I felt uncomfortable talking to him, sensing that he was pressing for an answer from me about what I was going to do, and I knew I hadn't come to the decision he preferred. But it was still my *life.*

You know, Kathy, I'd really like to see you pack up and leave for 6 months or so, get out and date other guys to see what's out there that you're missing. You've got to find some meaning for your life, and it certainly isn't coming where you are now! At least you're not pregnant.

Yeah. Maybe I should leave for awhile and give Ted a chance to get his act together.

Is there any place you can go?

Well, I'm not running home, if that's what you mean. That's living with the failure. There are people on the west coast, but I'd rather just grab the dogs and be a ski bum—get lost in the mountains.

I don't think being alone is what you need right now. *He and Miriam were in agreement on that one, but they weren't the ones to endure the pain of leaving. I would have to, and I knew I couldn't, no matter what I was saying to the contrary.*

Any Other Song

Since I was so unsettled about what to do with my marriage, I went with Darley and Kelly to Friday Afternoon Club that afternoon. That was the night I had arranged to meet Steve, but I deliberately suggested we go any place other than where we might coincidentally run into him. I left a note for Ted giving him a general idea of where I was; unfortunately he showed up to escort me home. Not in the mood to be alone with him, I suggested a compromise—I stayed and he took the pills. Nice gesture.

Hours later, after having hit the major singles bars, we were drunk enough to do anything. We'd met some guys who bought a few rounds, then one of them suggested he take me home. I laughed when he said it didn't matter that I was married. But the nightmare I created two months before came screaming back to me, and I coolly declined his offer. Darley and Kelly deposited me back at the apartment; it was 3:00, and Ted was awake enough to demand to know where I'd been. In disgust, he moved to the spare room. Fine. I was too tired anyway.

The rest of the weekend, whenever I wasn't doing something that required my full attention, I dwelled on how best to get it over with. I couldn't even concentrate on Sunday's sermon, and mused at the ease of appearing attentive while letting my imagination soar. No one made any good arguments as to why I should keep on going. Of all the alternatives—suicide, separation, or stagnation—the first looked the best. In preparation, I was able to have my skis fixed Saturday so that when the season opened the next week, I'd be ready. Sort of mix it up, and take off down the slope, making it look like an unfortunate accident.

Saturday evening I invited everyone over for dinner to combine a celebration for Lindy's sister's birthday and a semi-housewarming. As I was whipping up dinner, both Jo and Lindy came in to ask how things were going. It was all I could do to keep from bursting out in tears about how utterly uptight and depressed I was. I continued to play my stoic game well enough to fool everyone who mattered. The part of me that made suicide logical had taken over, and inside I cried. Even Nance, who stayed late that night to talk with Ted and me, had no idea what was happening. I honestly thought no one cared enough to really dig and find out. It wasn't worth their time and effort.

Ted was on call again Sunday, so Lindy invited me next door to talk. Snow began to fall outside as I walked over in the silence. I think having the three of them as neighbors—Nancy, Lindy and Jo—sort of made me feel safer. While Lindy finished washing her dishes, I vaguely alluded to my sense of being on the brink.

E. J. Daniel

Kathy, if you don't open up and tell Ted and Dr. Westberg how serious you are about all of this, as soon as you see them, I won't believe you really want help!

They know I'm serious, and nothing's happened! What about Labor Day? How many ways do I have to tell people?

You have to specifically tell them you fully intend to kill yourself by skiing into a tree. Then, if they don't hospitalize you, it's on their heads. Just promise me, *please,* that you'll come and get me before it's too late, and Nance and I will take you to the hospital. *She seemed coldly professional, and it frightened me. But the serious tone didn't impress me long enough to make me change my mind about dying. It was simply a matter of when.*

As I stumbled back to my apartment in the blowing snow, I barely noticed the encroaching blizzard. What's one more storm amid crushed snow drifts and stale yellow sunshine of a wasted November?

It had been a month since Ted and I saw Dr. Westberg, and we grudgingly kept our appointment Tuesday afternoon. We had already had one argument, and walked to his office in icy silence. He responded rather somberly to our morose condition.

Well! I can see things aren't progressing too smoothly. This is the worst I think I've ever seen you two. *What an opening comment for us to begin spontaneous, soul-searching commentaries on our sad states of mind. Neither of us was in the mood for talking, and after 45 minutes of dragged out semiconversation, he suggested we see him separately.*

Dr. Westberg didn't seem to take my suicidal intent more seriously than to arrange to see me again the next morning. Ted was in a mild state of shock with the news-break, but I chose to ignore him; he was supposed to see Westberg the following Monday, after Thanksgiving. I left Ted to finish playing student at the hospital, disregarding his vow to not let me go skiing, and plodded home to plan the best time. The wind was bitter cold, and I concluded that it didn't really matter if I never saw Monday. They weren't powerful enough to keep me from doing what I wanted.

When I got home, the phone was ringing. It was the animal shelter, claiming they'd picked up one of our dogs. He'd been hit by a truck, sustaining a concussion, fractured hip, and crushed shoulder, and they wanted permission to put him to sleep. If only I'd pushed for moving into a place with a fenced yard. It was my fault he'd gotten out; I'd killed my pup! There was now no other door.

Westberg and I met again Wednesday morning; he did more talking at that visit than in all of the previous sessions combined,

Any Other Song

taking advantage of my acutely depressed silence. But I bristled when I heard him saying how unfortunate it was that I had aligned myself with the proponents of the now-defunct custom of making a marriage last.

. . . Society has changed, and you need to see separation as a viable alternative to killing yourself. That certainly must be the lesser sin of the two. I don't believe that Christianity condones suicide! And at 24, your life is hardly washed up. There are other jobs you can apply for, other places to live. You need to see positive alternatives before you can start being happy again. What gibberish! He was wrong, all wrong. I knew that so clearly it surprised me. Unfortunate for him that he didn't understand me. Unfortunate for me that I'd been unable to show him how fantastic knowing God was. Not in a position to counter his summation, I said nothing.

You're not appearing to enjoy this depression you're in.

Oh, on the contrary! I love *being depressed.*

Do you need more pills, Kathy? What?

I hesitated slightly before nodding my head. He was so dumb I couldn't believe it! I'd found the way out, and was happy to add to my already large hoard. I raced to the pharmacy to fill my new prescription before returning to work.

There was a party in our lab that afternoon, and in anticipation I gulped a couple of beers at lunch with matching handfulls of blue pills. An appropriate beginning. As the get-together gained momentum, I paired handfulls with each cup of wine. It wasn't enough yet to really do anything, but I still had plenty of time and pills. I jumped when one of our docs motioned me into the hallway to talk.

Kathy. You know that Ted has been taking this pretty hard. You really need to stick by him. If you want this marriage to work, you should stay and get him to drop out of school for awhile, so he can sort out his priorities. School's just relentless. *Rob was unusually blunt. Ted was obviously talking to someone, after all. But I was sick of that song and dance.*

Uh, did he tell you what sort of problems there were?

He said you had suicidal tendencies. *I almost burst out laughing. Somehow I'd lost the audience; like the play had been going on for several hours when the crowd finally showed up, ignorant that they'd missed anything.*

Well, thanks for caring enough to tell me that. I'll sure work on it. *He smiled and turned away from me. I fumbled back into the lab, gulping another handful of the tiny blue pills that slid so easily down my lumpy throat. No one cared, really, you know, so why should I?*

E. J. Daniel

I hated everyone for their togetherness when I was so alone, hated everything for being the way it was and not the way I wanted it, hated myself for being such a failure—utterly, completely.

By the time I staggered home, I barely remembered my promise to Lindy. Inside I decided to drop by her apartment just to see if she was around. Jo answered the door, and I couldn't figure out what to do or say, as I didn't want to involve her in any more of my garbage. It wasn't fair to get her involved. We were casually visiting when Lindy finally came home. I tossed an empty pill vial to her; she plopped heavily onto the couch and just stared at me.

How many have you taken?

Around fifty. *Jo was watching us in horror.*

Is this a game?

No, this is not a game Lindy! *Storming out of her apartment into the snow, I exploded into my bathroom to finish off the remaining pills and everything else I could find. A game! I'm just really sure. Just as I turned out the bathroom light, careful to avoid looking at myself in the mirror, Jo and Lindy walked into the living room.*

Kathy, I want you to go with Lindy to the Emergency Room right now, if you're serious about asking for help.

If I'm serious? I backed into the hallway, away from them, fearful of the consequences of going, but their expressions said I'd better go anyway. At that moment, I cared more for what they thought of me than how totally worthless I felt. But I hated myself for having told them.

Reluctantly, I put on my coat and slowly walked with Lindy to the ER.

What happened today that set you off? What was going on? Why? . . . *I didn't know. My head was spinning as we wound our way through the frozen sections of snow. She was in a bigger hurry to get there than I was, leading the way. Abruptly she stopped.*

You know, Kathy. It'd be easier to help you if you didn't kick and scream in protest. *She was right.*

But as soon as we were inside the heavy glass and steel doors, I wanted to turn around and run. Before I could take any evasive action, she hustled me back to Emergency Psychiatry. My time was running out.

Lindy, what would you say if I just left?

She looked pensively at me, and I couldn't believe all of the pain and hurt I saw in her tired eyes. Surely I hadn't done that to her, had I? Not me.

I could do one of two things—either chase after you, but that's al-

Any Other Song

ways a game, or I could wait for you to show up comatose somewhere. But I'd be more inclined to follow you because I couldn't stand not knowing where you were. I'd just like to see you up on 8 East, in a protected environment. Ok? Please, Kath . . . *What had I done?*

Lindy gathered herself together and left me alone to vegetate in the carpeted room. She was on call, and promised she'd be back. My dizziness was rapidly deepening when Dr. Westberg strolled in.

Well, Kathy. Hello. What happened? *What does it look like? Lindy made me promise to tell him how what he'd said that morning made me angry enough to precipitate the supposed overdose. This was cutting into his suppertime.*

How many pills have you taken, and how long ago?

Around 80 of the Stelazine, and 40 or more aspirin, starting a little after our session this morning. *Things were getting very slow and muddy, and I couldn't tell if what I meant to say came out meaning the same. Must have been the wine.*

I guess I pushed you too hard this morning, but you should have told me how you were feeling. You know we'll have to pump you out. Are your ears ringing?

I nodded, but was planning to bolt as soon as he disappeared. I didn't want to be pumped out. Whatever that involved. Certainly there must be other ways of handling overdoses. But before I could muster up the momentum to fade out of the hospital, Dr. Westberg came back followed by a short, blue-smocked nurse. I began to panic as she escorted me back to the too-familiar Emergency Room.

How many pills have you taken? *She didn't sound concerned.*

Not enough. *Dr. Westberg mumbled he'd be back later as we walked into the booth.*

First I need to take your vitals. Ok? Sit up here on the stretcher for me. *I tried to follow what she was saying, having trouble thinking clearly. But even in my drugged state, I noted her mechanical power trip as she scribbled on a corner of the papered bed:* 130/80, 100. Now. Strip to the waist and put this gown on. We're going to have to wash all those pills out. *She turned to close the curtains while I just sat there, wondering what to do next. I must have looked a little uncooperative to her when she turned around and saw I hadn't moved. I was thinking I didn't want to be there.*

Look! There's enough junk inside to *kill* you! Do you understand? Now, come on. I'll help you.

The whole idea was to take enough to be fatal, so it must have only been the way she said it that scared me. Obediently I stripped down and put on the thin blue gown as another nurse, taller and dusty blonde, whisked in kicking a pail in front of her and dragging an IV stand rigged for lavage. The lights were too bright, their uniforms too intensely blue and yellow, my head too slow.

Just lie down on your back for now. We have to draw some blood and get this IV started first. *These weren't nurses, they were computers, over-programmed, so that I felt something more than detestable. Maybe they didn't like ODs, but that didn't mean they had to be so bitchy about it all. Maybe their lives made sense. Maybe they were happy doing purposeful things, but that just wasn't true for me! And why couldn't I just quit when my life stopped working? Why did I have to go through all of this spiteful treatment? Where was everyone who said they'd cared? Those-in-blue let me know how repulsive I was by missing my vein for the IV four times, finally securing it with a roll of tape so it would hold. If they were trying to make me hurt for what I'd done, they were succeeding gloriously. The shorter nurse left to help with another overdose, so Brenda finished setting the equipment up.*

Ok. I want you to swallow this tube just like you would drink a coke. *She'd swabbed something like vaseline all over the end of a huge clear garden hose, and before I could even think, tried jamming it down my throat. I jerked my head away in alarm, shoving the tube away from my mouth. Brenda turned grotesquely livid.*

Look! You can either help me with this, or I'll strap you down and force it down your throat! You came here for help, and we're going to treat you, one way or another! Which is it going to be?

A nurse must have overheard her explosion, and hurried in to help push the side of my head into the stretcher padding as Brenda poked the plastic tube down my throat into my stomach. It was degrading, and inside I cried in terror. Just keep swallowing. That's it. Breathe through your mouth.

I kept gagging in panic, especially when I saw the bloody secretions dribbling from my mouth into the emesis basin. Take deep breaths through your mouth, and stop biting the tube. If you'd relax, it would go much easier. Now, keep lying on your side while I hook the rest of this up. *Julie left once things were under control, and I watched in gothic horror as Brenda began to flood my stomach with the solution that had been suspended next to the slowly dripping IV bag. She reclamped one tube and drained off my stomach, the contents emptying noisily into the pail on the floor. At least I hadn't eaten all day.*

Westberg dropped by in the middle of the dehumanization. What have you gotten?

Oh, a bunch of blue pills, and I guess some aspirin tabs, right at first.

Any Other Song

Good. You got the Stelazine. *He smirked as he sauntered out. Gooey drool oozed out my gawking mouth, reeking of wine, as the dousing of liter after liter of tap water continued, sloshing in and out of my stomach. I couldn't stand it any longer, and tried to mumble around the hose that I'd had enough.*

Brenda looked down at me, cold and unfeeling. We're only about a third of the way through. Now keep your arm out of the way or you'll pull out your IV. Just keep taking deep breaths and you'll be just fine. *Like shit! If only I'd waited a little longer, those-in-white couldn't have done this to me, or at least I wouldn't have noticed it as much—or could've been dead. Where was Lindy? Why had I even come in with her, anyway?*

The curtains hadn't been completely closed, and anyone and everyone walking by peered in, adding to my humiliation. I tried staring at everything but Brenda and the gaggy network of tubes in an attempt to keep my mind off the nauseating trauma.

Alright. I have to put some medicine down you. Try not to gag on it, because you really need to keep this down. *I'd never heard of any medicine that was pitch black! It felt like she'd been flushing me out for hours. She hooked up a huge syringe to the end of the lavage hose, poured the black syrup in and pumped it down the tube inside me. The thought of that tar going down my throat into my stomach was more repulsive than the gurgling sensation of lavage.* I'll be back in a couple of minutes. Don't move!

The shorter nurse had stuck her head in to see if things were progressing smoothly enough for Brenda to leave and help her with the other OD. That made me angry. For some reason I'd thought I was the only one who could call it quits. At least, only one per night per ER, please; I needed to be a special case. Maybe that explained the nurses' complete disgust, not that it justified their aloofness.

After she'd been gone for a lot longer than several minutes, I panicked over all the saliva filling up in my throat around the tube, making it nearly impossible to breathe. How appropriate to spend all of that energy pumping out my stomach only to have me choke to death because I'd been left alone too long to aspirate on my spit. I couldn't decide between making enough noise to attract attention to my deserted body or remaining immovable as ordered. Hoping to calm my breathing, I closed my eyes, praying someone would come.

Looks like you got your punishment for the overdose! *Of all the people I did not want to see, Ted showed up. I can't believe how mad*

I am at you! You know God's angry for what you did. Aren't you just hating yourself for this? All ER staff despise people who attempt suicide. Medicine is devoted to saving lives and people like you destroy it. *Oh, Jesus—why did You let him find me?*

I couldn't even talk back, and he took advantage of it. I would've ripped the tube out myself at that point, but I was afraid that it would make me aspirate in the process. Strange I should be afraid.

Just then a doc, black bag in hand, stuck his head in the room, and I finally communicated to him that I desperately wanted the tar-filled tube out. At least he obliged me, ending the initial nightmare. I lay there numb, ears pounding.

I need to do a physical on you. Are your ears still ringing? *I nodded, hardly all together. He was short, and smelled like those spicy herb teas (must have been torn away from supper to do this exam). Ted continued to sit zombie-like in the corner of the tiny cubicle, seeming not to appreciate the doc's routine assessment. Big deal.*

> Progress note: 24-year-old female known well to Dr. Westberg, psychiatrist, with history of suicide attempt in past—by lacerating wrists. Today beginning at 1 PM while drinking wine, taking Bufferin and Stelazine (which she has been taking on regular basis now a short time), taking 80 2mg Stelazine between 1–5 PM and 40 tabs Bufferin at approximately 5 PM. At this time has tinnitus without shortness of breath, dizziness, or syncope. No nausea or vomiting, gastric irritation or diarrhea. Alert, cooperative, clear speech. As per psychiatry, will be admitted to psych ward per Dr. Westberg.

After the family practitioner resident had completed his cursory exam, Brenda came back in. Guess what? I have to draw more blood. We need to check and see that your aspirin level's going down and not up. When the results get back, if everything's Ok, they'll take you upstairs. *Upstairs?* I also need to change your IV. This one's running too slow, and we need to get another bag inside you. *Ramrod medicine.*

Ted's presence continued to make me wish that I'd succeeded at the attempt. I wanted him to leave—forever—but he insisted on hanging around, probably thinking he was lending me moral support or something asinine like that. I just ignored him. Dr. Westberg interrupted to say good-bye before fleeing to the mountains for a long weekend of skiing.

We're going to keep you upstairs for a few days and I'll see you on Monday when I get back. Are your ears still ringing? *I nodded. Wednesday to Monday sounded longer than a few days, but I was too groggy to protest. I needed to find a bathroom, but couldn't find a*

Any Other Song

nurse to help. I thought those test results would never get reported, I'd never be able to leave, Ted would never go home. I wanted to die so badly or to at least cry, but I was too used up to do anything but stare at the curtains.

Kathy. You can get dressed now. They're here to take you upstairs. Even though Julie was the nurse who'd helped Brenda jab down that terrible tube, she was warmly mellow as she gently removed the patchwork tape from the poorly done IV. I wondered what kept her going when I wanted so fiercely to die.

Admitting note: 24-year-old wife of 3rd year med student brought in by friend after ingesting 40 ASA and 60 2mg Stelazine with unknown amount of ethyl alcohol approximately 20 minutes before coming to ER and 8 hours after a session with me. She states that she is sorry that she did not kill herself and remains highly suicidal. The history was given in a withdrawn, sullen and angry manner. After the session today patient felt that I didn't understand her moral dilemma about separating from husband and took the Stelazine that I gave her plus others that she had at home. Eventually she called a friend who brought her in. I first saw patient and husband last March for 4 sessions after patient was hospitalized here in neurology for encephalitis following 3 days of headaches—lumbar puncture, scan and angiogram were within normal limits. At that time, there was marital discord. However, things settled down after about one month. I saw them again for 4 sessions in October after patient called Dr. Reilley on overdose one month before. Since then patient has made multiple threats and some gestures usually when someone doesn't understand her. The dilemma is that she wants to separate but can't because of shame and fundamentalist Christianity. Furthermore, patient believes that Satan may be involved. Her present solution (besides suicide) is talking with Miriam Guest, a Christian marriage therapist. However, patient feels that she can't reach the ideals of a "good" wife and resents terribly her husband's school, etc. Patient has made previous suicide gestures—once at age 17 after fight with father. At present she feels lonely, distant, angry and misunderstood. My alliance with her is nonexistent. It is somewhat better with Dr. Reilley and Mrs. Guest. The problem with her relationship with me is: 1) my Thanksgiving vacation, 2) that I suggested a trial separation. While I acknowledged that this would be difficult, apparently it was not enough. Another problem is that the more understanding and empathetic people are, the more frightened and isolated she feels. At present, shows no psychotic symptoms, is groggy from OD and has tinnitus. Remains at suicide risk. Plan is to continue to try to establish a therapeutic relationship and explore the possibilities of separation and a return to parents. She should not be allowed off the ward unattended and she should be closely observed on the ward. She should not be allowed to leave under any circumstances. After she recovers from OD, Stelazine 2 mg q 4 hours as needed should be available for "panicky feeling." I will be at 299-8855 until Thursday PM and then at 1-770-3004 until Monday AM.

TEN

and the next morning
you wish desperately
it was only a
nightmare.
It never really happened—
not to me.
Maybe,
maybe to a part
of me.
But i didn't
overdose.
That's not me.
Not now—
NOT EVER.

and the cage
those-in-white
put me in
behind locked doors and
steel-mesh screens
in a façade of
brighter oranges and greens
made me wish
there was someone,
anyone,
to cry to

Any Other Song

> *melting away the
> deeper pain and hurt
> of what i had done.*

The snow continued to fall in gentle gusts of early winter wind. I stared out at a morning I never expected to wake up to. Inside, there were blue carpets and fresh, multicolored walls, plants in the hallway and dayroom, and roll-away beds covered in rich Herculon plaids. But I was still on a psychiatric floor, on suicide precaution, restricted to the ward. That fact, plus the anger I felt at having been grilled by one of the male staff (concerning why, when, how much, how I got along with my father, and other Freudian crap), kept me awake off and on all night, aided by the continual checking of the staff. They let me crash at 11:30, finally, after an additional quizzing by the on-call shrink. No one had bothered to show me where blankets, towels or anything else were, and I hadn't exactly come prepared to spend the night. It was appropriate, though, after the way I'd been treated in the Emergency Room. I just assumed it was additional punishment. I also resented the feeling that Lindy had deserted me. That was fine—I didn't deserve her, anyway.

For lack of anything else to do that morning, I dressed early, and sat curled up in a corner of the bed, waiting, scared. The same small blonde nurse who'd stopped to check on me at 4 AM to avert my soaring temp, interrupted my withdrawal.

Well, good morning! I'm Cory, and your breakfast is down the hall. Have you been shown around yet?

I wasn't talkative, to say the least, and was still terribly hung over. Silently, I wandered around with her to see what protective environment Lindy had coaxed me into, of locked doors and heavily screened windows. In the dayroom I was introduced to several other inmates eating breakfast in orderly fashion, except for one obviously retarded kid whose food lay scattered on the floor around his chair. Certainly a motley conglomeration of battered humanity.

Later, Ted brought me some clothes and things for the duration, in spite of his acute anger over what I'd done, which I couldn't divorce from a rage at me. I painfully endured the hurt in his eyes, finally begging him to just leave.

After the token Thanksgiving dinner, in the midst of football, I was surprised by a visit from our Pastor. It was nice to know that he cared enough to disrupt his family's holiday celebration, but I had difficulty concentrating on what he was saying, mostly because I felt so horrible.

You know, Kathy, you fight and fight to have your own way, but the Lord just isn't going to let you go. I think that's really something to be thankful for! *I don't remember his saying much of anything else, and I didn't have any response for even that. What do you say? What else could he do?*

The remainder of the day passed in a shaky haze, my mind and body ravaged from the invasive procedure of Wednesday and the leftover absorbed pills. I remained secluded in my room at the end of the hall, and was checked on every hour or so by the motley staff.

> Promises
> he gave to you
> of dreams-to-come-true
> some magic noon
> and sunrises, too,
> balloons and kisses
> and little girl wishes,
> any fantasy,
> he said, but—
> maybe
> next year. . .

Friday morning the night nurse came in to check on me again before going home. Khyra assured me that suicide was almost impossible on the ward, and being on suicide precautions would hopefully eliminate any other slim chances. That was an interesting topic to be chatting about. Maybe with her M.S. in psych nursing she thought we could be strictly objective about a subjective area. But it doesn't work that way. Her comment just made me dwell on dying even more.

In the afternoon, Dr. Reilley came up to see me—concerned, but not surprised that I was there. Word gets around.

On Saturday, I decided to hang myself from the bathroom door with my oversized football jersey. I was going to make them all sorry I'd been admitted. The lights were out in my room that evening, and I sat staring at my handmade noose which hung against the door. The noose glowed slightly from the parking lot lights gleaming eight flights below. The rust painted room was quietly comfortable, and thoughts about death floated easily through my mind. But I prayed that if I wasn't supposed to die then, that some-

Any Other Song

one would come and stop me, or find me before it was too late. But no one would. Why should they? And I started crying in remorse. I was standing on the small white table I'd propped next to the door, trying to put the noose over my head, when I heard Ted's voice in the hallway. My heart jumped into my throat and I quietly hopped down and crouched in the darkened corner to hide. If I was to be found, I did not want him to do the finding. The absence of light must have made him think I wasn't in the room, and he soon left me to my suicidal contemplations. Withdrawn protectively into a ball in the small space, I was nearly hyperventilating as I envisioned my body suspended lifeless from the cloth noose.

Kathy? Oh! You scared me! A gentle nurse had discovered me crouched in the peaceful darkness. I was unable to say anything, but heard Ted's voice boom outside.

Can't I come in?

No! Wait there, please! The lights were still off.

Why can't I come in and see my wife? I'm going to come in!

No! Just wait out in the hall, please! She shut the door in his face, and came over to sit on the floor directly in front of me. *What's happening, Kathy?* Her Texas accent was soft as she rested her hand on my pulled-up knees. She said nothing about the conspicuous noose just visible in the twilight. There was only an eerie silence.

She waited awhile before taking my hand and urging me up out of my protected corner. Wonderful first impression I'd made. *How about if I stay with you while you talk with your husband? I know this isn't the best of times, but you only need to see him for a short while, Ok?*

I could only nod. The last thing in the world I was in the mood for was conversation with Ted after having decided to give up. At least he didn't stay long, uncomfortable with Jude being in on his pressuring comments, and left us alone to talk.

Hey, Kath. I kind of know how hard it is! My husband's a doc; we were married his senior year of med school. It's just that when things like their time commitment get in the way, you can't feel it's the end of the world! You've got a lot more to offer than that—believe me! She didn't know me. I listened, but inside couldn't accept it as true for me. *I wish I could be around to help you more, but I'm only part-time.* That figured. I stared at the floor, angry that God had answered my half-hearted prayer. Jude was the only one who'd cared enough to find me, but with her leaving it was just another thing that started out too good to be true, and then was quickly taken away. *If you think I can help, call me at home. Really!*

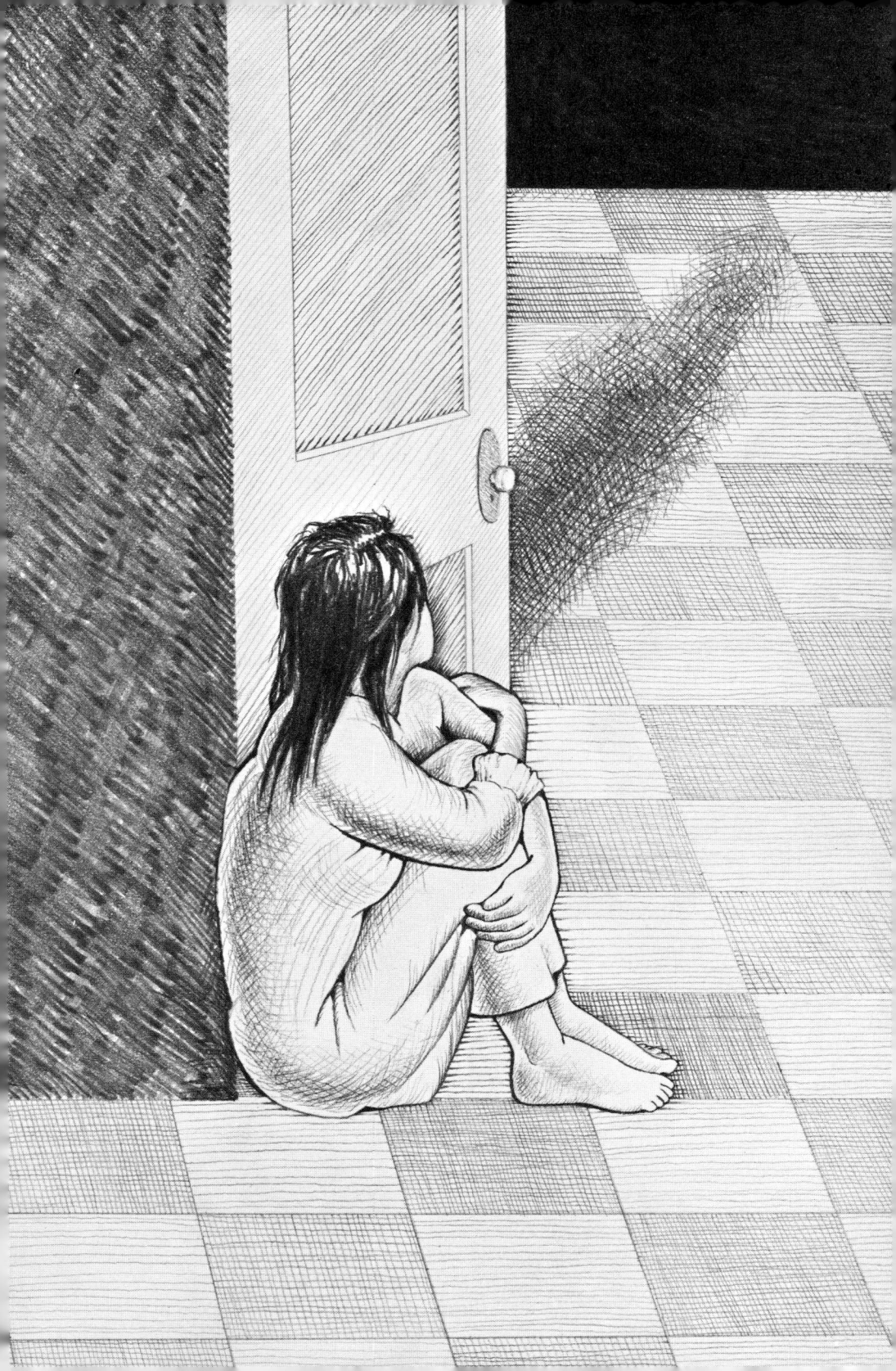

E. J. Daniel

I looked at Jude and halfway laughed. That one I'd heard before. But I didn't blame BJ for giving up—who wouldn't with someone who couldn't put into practice all the loving advice she'd freely given? I didn't blame anyone for giving up on me, leaving, not being there, whatever. I was supposed to be the strong, together person, and if I'd given up on myself, everyone else should have long ago. Especially God.

> to hate
> that which God
> lovingly created
> when hope was warm and
> light was understanding until
> evening edged inside
> fogging His reason
> for allowing grief
> over some not-so-distant sins that
> haunt in shadowed webs
> of a house once swept free
> but now too cluttered with confusion—
> to hate that
> is to
> destroy
> my
> self.

Sunday was sadder. It was only a piece of me that was hospitalized; the rest of me had already died, and Sunday I was in mourning. And they kept me on suicide precautions, while the other patients roamed free. I lost track of the endless hours that persisted into days.

> "best of both worlds," they say, and
> "jack of all trades"—come
> one, come all! See how she
> walks and falls
> death-defying acts (all
> without success)
> photographer-musician-cook
> maker-of-love (not babies)
> "master of none"
> (including
> dy-
> ing).

I couldn't find the energy to go through with another hanging attempt.

Any Other Song

 Mom panicked from Ted's long-distance call of alarm, and flew in, completely ruining her holiday. He must have cabled everyone he knew to tell them the terrible news—Kathy's finally cracked! She was very upset that I didn't go all out to welcome her; she didn't understand that I didn't want to see the very people who were so hurt and disappointed by my failure to cope. After a stormy family meeting on Monday, where I was told to be completely open and honest (which went over like an atomic blast while my sister watched in agonizing disbelief), Mom announced she was leaving the next day, *"if that's how you feel!"* She and Ted were both stunned by my angry outbursts during the meeting, and explicitly let me know how unfeeling I was.
 I'd only been in the hospital five calendar days, and the staff continued to check on me regularly. It seemed less harsh now. Old patients left, hardly noticed, and newer, stranger ones were admitted, transforming it into a geriatrics ward. I never belonged there in the first place. So to make room for an older male alcoholic, I was moved out of my comfortable solitude into a yellow room already occupied by a 20-year-old girl who had attempted suicide by gas. I don't know what their intent was, but I finally couldn't tolerate her rummaging through my personal effects.
 Cassandra! If you don't stay out of my things and shut your foul mouth, I'm gonna punch you out! That was an unfortunate threat I uttered out of impatience, and never intended to have to back up. But her morning dullness and general distaste for her new roommate quickly escalated into uncontrolled fury. Aside from the garbage that spewed out of her mouth, she bombarded me with kicks, knee jabs and punches to my face and head. I tried grabbing her flailing arms, but soon gave up and ran out of the room in shock, regretting I'd chosen to vent my frustration on her.
 Hey! Can someone calm Cassandra down? She's a little out of control! She chased me down the hall, screaming.
 They soon calmed her down, and then they wanted an explanation. *What happened, Kathy? She's never done that before.* I made some excuse. In spite of that confrontation, though, I would rather have roomed with Cass than with the middle-aged teacher waging a legal battle to get discharged. She'd "mistakenly" taken too many tranquilizers. After a couple of days she got out, but she had found time before she left to accuse me of playing a game with the staff. "I can see right through you." That a social studies teacher could be such an expert in psychology was amazing.
 Tuesday night the five of us still left were given special pass privi-

leges to get a real pizza—out of the hospital. Those-in-white gave the others strict orders to watch me, as I didn't have off-grounds privileges. I think the staff was just tired of the responsibility.

Ecstatically we trucked across the street, feeling so free! We gorged on pizza, guzzled two pitchers of beer and seemed to be handling our freedom calmly, when Lynne suddenly became extremely anxious. Burly-bearded John (in for a drinking problem) walked her back to the hospital door, and rejoined us with a few six-packs on our way to Margy's apartment. By then it was well after 10:00. John called back to the ward to let them know we were only having a little party, but they weren't too pleased, and wanted us back in an hour. We were ready to go back after a few more beers, a joint and boogieing that irritated the tenants. They almost called the police; that would have been sticky.

Back on the floor, the staff's disappointment was blatant, and they blamed John and me that Margy was falling apart. Too many beers, too much grass. The three of us clung to each other in the middle of the floor, trying to calm her. She wanted nothing to do with Peppermint Patty and Jack the Ripper.

You two have no business helping Margy! You are patients, not staff. So let us take care of her and you go on to bed! *I was infuriated! I bolted down an adjoining hallway, plopping down in the darkness to try and calm down. Out of sheer stupidity, Jack followed me and attempted to talk with me. Without saying a word, I glared up at him and left the jerk staring at the floor where I'd been sitting.*

I went back to Margy, finally quieted by Khyra. We got her into bed and she was still clutching my hand. I felt that maybe I wasn't as out of control as it seemed, even though I didn't have any answers for her—not after what I'd done and where I was. And I couldn't understand why "out there" people destroy such fragile, sensitive people as Margy.

On my way back to my room John met me with a hug that communicated everything a hug could under those circumstances, in that place, so late at night. I even apologized to Peppermint before she went home.

I'm sorry I blew it, but at least I didn't split. *I wished I had, but she didn't hear that.*

The icy reality
of being left alone
is worsened
when it's inside

Any Other Song

*tearing
at my sensitivity
to another's pain—
or maybe my own.*

*It's as though
i was a piece of of fragile coral left
exposed on the sun-hot beach
after the tide roared out, foaming green,
leaving me a broken orange heap.*

*Maybe the roots are still there
but the most important parts of me
are lost and i wait in
terror
for the tide to surge back
drowning and scattering
the remaining fractured shards
forever.*

ELEVEN

One week after I'd been hospitalized, the suicide precautions were dropped, supposedly as a result of the responsibility shown on the Tuesday night pass. No one explained the change to me. Those-in-white just presumed I was ready. No one seemed to understand what was going on inside. I wasn't able to make them hear what I was really saying . . .

> Those-in-white and others
> say i'm only
> playing a game,
> that i really know
> who i am and
> where.
> They don't hear
> what i'm saying
> or believe my angry threats.
> They think they see
> me inside
> but they're misreading
> my distorted outside.
> i've tried
> to tell them
> to show them
> that it's not
> a game

Any Other Song

> and that i need their
> help and
> loving understanding
> to find a way
> back to that part of me
> that is fighting desperately for—
> what was that again?

Jude was gone and no one heard me. There were too many goal meetings of drawn-out disillusionments, too many small groups of petty accusations, empty daily chats with passive shrinks, and irregular ventilations with the frantically busy nursing staff. On one of the rare occasions when Lindy found me, Nance was visiting. As we sat out in the hall talking, just the three of us, for a second it was as though we weren't really there, and could have been back on our October trip enjoying each other's company, cruising in a mellow autumn afternoon. But their deeply concerned faces made that fantasy dissipate into agony.

> Friday night I drifted in dreams of lying on a windswept, bleached ivory beach—a too-hot fireball finally breaking through a blue, comfortable fog, in the shelter of sea-worn boulders etched with cherished yesterdays in a too-intense present, tears oozing between fissures. Gulls strutted atop barnacled rocks, peering curiously at me, yet not deserting the sobbing. Buckbrush and rusted salt cedar shielded me from the blistering off-shore gusts, while the droning green surf lulled away my loneliness.

The longer I was hospitalized, the more it seemed that I was increasingly tired and apathetic, rather than pulled together. I didn't understand why I wanted those who meant so much to me to come by, but was embarrassed and withdrawn while they were there. When Miriam came to see me, I thought I would be violently ill from anxiety. I'd totally failed her, and just couldn't bear having her see me there, hearing about how God loved me anyway, because it didn't make any sense. Dr. Westberg had called her the day it'd happened.

So how are you doing, Kathy?

I looked everywhere but at her. *As well as can be expected, I suppose. There's not really anything to do around here—play cards, ping pong, plunk the piano.* How she could tolerate spending time with me was beyond comprehension.

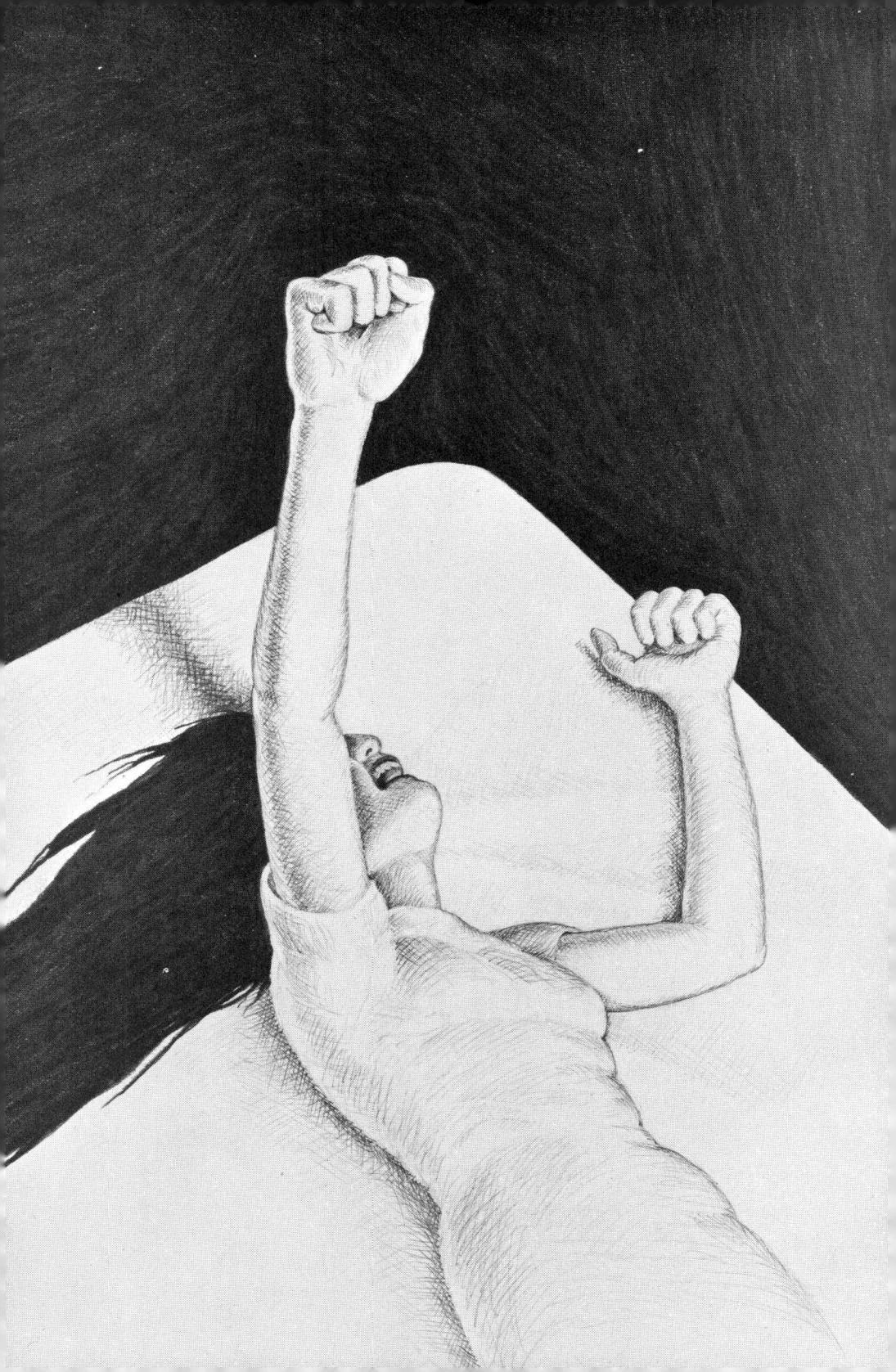

E. J. Daniel

Have you been reading from the Bible? *Did I even believe God cared I was there?*

Probably not as much as I should, but it just doesn't seem to help! I know in my head that God's still running the show, but that doesn't make it real to me. And He's never going to want to use me now, not after all this! I've lost everything saleable; there's nothing left of me to give! So, why doesn't He just let me go so I won't hurt anymore?

I'm really sorry you feel that way, Kathy. Trust me that there will come a time when you'll see that there is indeed much left for you to give. It took at least a year to get where you are now, and you can expect another year to get back. Don't be so hard on yourself. *With my mind, which Miriam said I wasn't using, I could understand what she was saying. But my feelings screamed out to be recognized, obliterating everything else. She left soon, uncomfortable with seeing me the way I was.*

Sunday afternoon Lindy and her sister visited me. Having them see me there made me ashamed; I couldn't accept where I was for the reasons that put me there because that wasn't in my script. No one had allowed for this blunder. It simply wasn't me and never should be. The tears I managed to keep inside ate away, but I couldn't open up. I'd dumped enough on Lindy already, and December was supposed to be happy.

Ted drifted by later to take me home on pass to visit my dog. He hadn't planned anything, but told the staff we were going out or something so they'd let him take me off the ward. I thought I could handle it adequately, but after a couple of hours at the apartment, I lost control of the inflating depression. In an intense state of panic, I was returned to the floor. As nonchalantly as I could, I suggested to Cory that I be put back on suicide precautions. She was actually grateful I'd told them how edgy I was, and she walked me down the hall to seclusion—four gray walls, no fixtures, and a blanket-covered mattress in the middle of the cold tile floor. Cory stayed with me for awhile, hoping to get me to cry or scream out my suppressed anger and hurt, but all I could do was cry. She gave me some Kleenex, and closed the door behind her as she left.

I couldn't let it out. I was afraid I'd break into a million pieces and no one would be able to put me back together. Maybe that was a reflection of how much, or how little, I trusted the staff. Maybe it showed to what extent I mistrusted myself. Or God. I don't know. But everything inside me groaned and begged to open up, desperate to be consoled and soothed, held and comforted, but it didn't happen.

Any Other Song

 Lou quietly stepped inside the dimmed room and sat down on the floor opposite me. She was the only other staff person who had tried to understand me, encouraging me to let it out, but still accepting when I couldn't. Kathy. I want you to roll over on your stomach and start pounding that mattress with your fists. Right now!
 I looked at her as though she was crazy. Lou, it's not going to work! It won't come out.
 Come on—try it! Start pounding. *I saw her weary face, and, hating myself, obediently began slugging the mattress.* Faster! Harder! *It felt terribly forced, but I kept at it until I collapsed, exhausted, face buried in the blanket.*
 Kathy—don't you see? We're trying to help, but you won't let us! *I groaned with silent deep sobs at having disappointed her. Chalk up one more failure.*
 A couple of weeks had floated past when I was moved to another ward, full privileges. I realized too late that I had been kept on suicide precaution for so long because those-in-white were genuinely concerned. The move was in preparation for discharge. That scared me, and on a Friday night pass with Ted, I drank myself into oblivion even though Cory had warned me not to drink because of the pills I was on. But I felt I couldn't cope without. Ted wouldn't bring me back when I first asked him to, thinking I was just a party-pooper, so I guzzled even more until he was convinced. Grudgingly, he dropped me off at the hospital and I staggered upstairs, alone, to a silent staff.

     Snow falls in the silent blue
      beyond my frosted
      locked windows
     as i question incessantly
   the once-purposeful moves i made
    resulting in my confinement
     behind such bars,
    cold and lonely in my
   self-perpetuated isolation.

    i grope for any shelter
    from a raging affect,
   finding only confusion
    with mere threads
   holding me intact.

E. J. Daniel

i quiver inside, breathless,
fearful of losing
those last delicate controls.

the wet, heavy snow
suffocates and smothers
the last of me
and i can't
get out from under it.

TWELVE

The Tuesday morning I was discharged I cried, but no one saw me. The security I originally resented had become my structured existence, and now I was having to say good-bye. There were people I wouldn't miss—like Frieda, who screamed and spit out profanity whenever she was put in seclusion. When those-in-white finally got her medically under control, she just wandered aimlessly in and out of the dayrooms mumbling, shooting wild-eyed glances at the patients. I wouldn't miss Debbie, who vegetated in her sheepshorn coat in any corner of the ward all day, staring blankly at the walls, with only an occasional smile for familiar staff that happened by. Nor would I miss the manic-depressive shrink. But when Lynne left the ward, it hurt. And Margy. We had grown to know each other in a special way, sharing things no one on the outside ever could. And most of all, John, because of his warm understanding. I had allowed a real attachment for them to develop that excluded those who'd never been where we were, and that made us closer—at least for the time we were there. It was a kind of strength, a defense against the criticism we suffered from people who couldn't begin to know how it feels.

The day before I left, Jude made a special trip to the hospital to sit in on my last family meeting. She seemed almost disappointed that I'd decided to go to the west coast to seek the counseling Ted

Any Other Song

had arranged. *Those-in-white didn't understand that I had to keep trying to make our marriage work, because I'd still be friends with and love unconditionally anyone else that was as close to me as Ted had been. So why not him? Hopefully, by getting away for awhile, I could clear my head and try to learn what was expected of me. No one in the hospital could fathom my responsibility to everyone I knew as a result of knowing the Lord. I just had to try every single avenue before I could consider separation a viable option.*

After the depressing session, Jude talked with me awhile before saying the good-byes I didn't want to hear. You're just like a battered child—someone who's been psychologically abused—and you've got to give yourself *time.* Please, if I can ever help, call me. And keep in touch while you're out there, because I want to know what's happening with you. *When she started crying, I saw that she was someone who cared enough. That's all I was asking for. But I feared I would always need more than anyone could give . . .*

> *show me you know*
> *and feel*
> *the same kind of pain*
> *in me, in you*
> *when good-byes are*
> *forever said,*
> *sometimes in tears.*
>
> *Tell me you care*
> *and love me*
> *regardless of things*
> *said and done,*
> *and that we'll be*
> *better people for*
> *having been here,*
> *unable to forget*
> *each other.*
>
> *Please, share with me*
> *at least in distant memory*
> *the tears and hurt*
> *opened in trust and*
> *promise that*
> *after the parting*
> *you'll still*
> *remember.*

Was it too much to ask? Maybe all anyone ever wants is to be known and remembered.

E. J. Daniel

Before my plane had even taken off, I was asking myself what I was doing. It seemed I'd spent all my life looking for someone special to care, and whenever I found someone, I would move or run away. I felt I never really mattered to anyone—at least not enough to make a noticeable difference in their lives or mine, and that was why, when my marriage stopped working, I quit trying. I lost patience trying to be what I thought I was supposed to be, and what everyone always expected me to be. In order to find some meaning, I looked everywhere I could. I found nothing in my relationship with Ted. And I felt prohibited from using the talents I thought were especially mine, in ways I'd always envisioned. I needed a purpose, a reason to keep trying even when there seemed to be nothing left of my life to make it worthwhile. I believed that the motivation had to come from someone else; it wasn't enough to try just for me, or just for Ted. I was nearly immobilized with an insatiable need to feel cared for in a special way, to be appreciated. Doing things for others had always given my life meaning, but when they stopped noticing, it all caved in. And if it didn't matter to anyone else, why should it matter to me?

my façade
should tell anyone
but
IT'S NOT WORKING
and no one sees
inside
how
IT'S NOT WORKING.
just a game
or nightmares
i never dreamed
nor wanted
since they've scarred me
forever
only
IT'S NOT WORKING.
the need to purge
such irony
by fire
tells everyone
IT'S NOT WORKING.

THIRTEEN

I had no idea what to expect when my plane landed, realizing that what might be offered there wouldn't be enough to fill the massive void I sensed mushrooming inside. I wasn't together enough to even know what I needed, or what it would take to get me to that point of knowing. Maybe I was just unable to actually tell anyone. But I had to try, somehow, at least once more, just to be sure that there might not still be a chance that I mattered to someone. That God might ask too much of me again, though, made me resentful of the bitter past He'd already allowed.

My parents were thrilled to see me, as Dr. Westberg accurately predicted, but overly cautious to not pressure me in any way. I hated it. It should have been totally different, because they weren't a conscious part of my frustration, and I didn't want to hurt them anymore. Mom took me to the private Christian counseling center that Jo had told Ted to get me involved with; she was hopeful they could patch up her deranged daughter. But it didn't work out; the counseling intern I talked with merely arranged for me to visit with the wife of a local surgeon. He must have thought the woman would be empathetic and of sufficient support to see me through the crisis. By then, though, I knew I needed more than friendly conversation.

I told Mom that Nance was scheduled to fly into the area to visit

Any Other Song

some friends on her way home for the holidays, and that she had invited me to come with her. *Mother was appalled I could even consider such an arrangement, and her shock reverberated loudly when Nance called from the airport.*

So how'd it go with the counseling? *Nance seemed to want it to work as much as Mom, but it wasn't to be. I told her of their patch-quilt efforts.*

Why don't you just fly down to L.A. with me on Saturday and see the people Miriam set you up with? Discuss it with your folks and I'll call you back tomorrow. Ok?

Gritting my teeth as I hung up the phone, I turned to face Mom, her eyes expectant. I hated her Pollyanna hope, her belief that it would all work out, because the rainbow just wasn't mine to find. Her "oh, sure—your father and I understand, but . . ." reasoning, uttered in such a way that I could only feel guilty for going with Nance, made me dread the pressure if I stayed. So I bought my ticket at the airport and left, unable to look back and wave.

On the plane, I tried not to think about what I was being shuffled into. I was just spending the weekend with Nance, a lull before the storm. We talked during the flight, on the way to her parent's house, and off and on through the night, working out each other's nightmares. I cherished every minute, wanting to stretch time into a dream I could feel comfortable in. After church on Sunday, I called Miriam to give her a status report of sorts: scared, Miriam. Hauntingly scared . . .

Monday Nance drove me out to the center, waiting outside the psychologist's office while I tried to be open and honest with this new therapist. I even shared my poetry, since I reportedly had such a difficult time speaking. Maybe he would hear me through my poems. The short, elfish, and incredibly gentle Ph.D. became engrossed in my creations.

Uh, Dr. Lander—may I have my friend come in now? *His pensive silence made me uncomfortable.*

Why don't we? I'd like to explain the situation to her. *I feared he was understanding me too well. His approach was more direct than Westberg's, certainly closer, but maybe that was because I was trying to trust him. Some tears even escaped, which never happened with Dr. Westberg. Nance poked her head in the doorway, giving me a "what's happening" look as she sat down across from me.*

Hello, Nancy. I'm Dr. Lander. Kathy tells me you're a medical student. *I stared at the rich oak coffee table stacked neatly with magazines and Kleenex.* Well, I think that the way things now stand, since we can't effectively take care of Kathy on an outpatient basis because of the travel involved, we should have her go back into the hospital for awhile. *A bomb. The reality of what was being arranged slowly sank in, and I couldn't stop the tears. I felt sick again, letting everyone down, especially Nance. She'd been so hopeful, so supportive, and I'd failed again.*

Nance quietly drove me home to get my clothes, and then on to the community hospital which, ironically, was only a few blocks from the big red brick church where I'd been baptized. On the unit, Nance and I waited somberly as the staff searched my belongings and checked me in. We slowly walked down to my four-bed room where she hugged me good-bye. Nance seemed as upset as I was when she left; then I was alone.

In a stupor I wandered down the hallway of the Christian Therapy Unit, past the nurses' station gleaming in the contrasting darkness.

Kathy! Hi. Would you like to talk awhile? *Turning around, I saw it was the soft nurse who had admitted me. Viv walked with me down to the comfortably dim reception area on the other side of the locked doors. I wasn't thinking very clearly through the Stelazine left over from that morning, plus their new drug regimen. It was hard to concentrate on what she said, but her gentle manner began to fill my void.*

Will you be on again tomorrow?

No, I'm only part-time. I'm sorry. But we'll talk again next time I'm on. Ok? *Good move, picking another seldom-there staff nurse to open up to.*

The next morning I was dragged abruptly out of my bed before breakfast for blood work. I didn't know why I was so groggy, and as the tech filled the last of six tubes, I became very lightheaded. Before I could say anything, I was gone . . .

I don't think she knows what's happened.

Kathy! Kathy, do you think you can get up now and change? Are you awake, Kathy?

My semialert body was slumped over in the chair, supported on either side by the night nurse and lab technician, who were wafting noxious ammonia under my nose. Then I became aware of my sopping wet nightgown. Just a little embarrassing.

Her eyes are Ok now.

Kathy, can you get up? It's alright. It happens all the time.

Apparently I still looked quite dazed, so they helped me into the

Any Other Song

bathroom to change while my two post-middle-aged roommates watched on in motherly concern. Those-in-white put my body back into bed. It was nothing to be ashamed of, they said—just an incorrect combination of medications. Psychiatric trial and error.

> Now that i am someplace
> where i never was,
> each Mellaril footstep echoes
> violently
> the Stelazine redundancy of
> being hospitalized
> in another attempt to
> piece together some Elavil remnants
> of an old used-up me that is
> only a Haldol shell,
> because something vacuumed out
> most of my insides
> that ever mattered,
> leaving only the Dalmane.
>
> Those-in-white have drugged me
> to the point that nothing matters—
> whether i'm whole or particled—
> and i'm saturated and scared
> of the Thorazine patients, the
> chipped and waxy bare walls and floors,
> and artificial help
> that doesn't help.

During one of the dull group sessions conducted by my new shrink, Dr. Rex, one of my roommates vehemently accused me of being a staff person incognito, planted purposely as a patient to get her upset enough to talk. I'd only been using a few of the psychological techniques I'd picked up in my other groups, but that incident created sufficient rift to move me out of that room to one across the hall. They'd just admitted a new patient, Rebekeh, who made life there much more bearable for me. A graduate student in chemistry, she'd admitted herself because she "hurt too bad inside"; I could identify with that. As she opened up, I tried to help her get things together because it made me feel there really might be something good and strong left in me if I could offer something to someone else. It was less painful concentrating on her problems, anyway; disregarding mine made coping possible, to the extent of denying there was even anything wrong. Since Rebekeh wasn't trusting the staff, I tabled my raging to give her some of my energy.

E. J. Daniel

*There are those who
care
when i care
if i'll just take the first step.*

*But i hesitate
from fear of rejection,
for getting close means
giving me. Yet
isn't it worth the price
to share deeply
with someone? Isn't that
what we're here for?*

*And i'll care
just as soon as i'm together
and give great gobs of me
to others who want it.
i've learned
what it is to love
unconditionally,
in spite of,
regardless of,
and how necessary it is to
pass it on.*

At the time, it made an incredible difference being hospitalized with other Christians. My mind comprehended that faith, along with many scriptural promises that drifted back demanding equal time with my errant emotions, but I still felt it was all too good to be true for me.

*seconds and minutes
and minutes and
hours and hours
and days and
months crawl by
as i wait for the
great disintegration
when afterward
i can enjoy and
treasure the life
that now is so
painfully unending.*

*yet i keep putting it off
fearing
that no one will be able to*

Any Other Song

*integrate me
into a
wholly peaceful person.*

*so when it happens,
promise me you'll
be there to lovingly
put the best pieces
into better places
than they were
and that tomorrow
you'll like me more
than i was before.*

One dusky evening I collapsed on my bed in sobs from the unbearable loneliness. Christmas came and went, barely celebrated, and Nance had returned to school. I was more alone than I'd ever felt possible. I even tried calling BJ to apologize for having dumped on her so many months before. After finding out where I was, she hung up, leaving me with the stabbing pain of knowing I had totally destroyed that warm relationship. The emptiness wouldn't quit nagging at me. Why hadn't God allowed me to die?

Hey, Kathy. What's wrong? I wanted to be held and comforted so badly, but my outside wouldn't allow it. Besides, I was supposed to be an adult and able to cope with pain. The rock, not some battered little girl. I fought the surging undercurrent that threatened to explode me into a million pieces, and remained tautly stretched out on the bed, burying endless tears in my pillow. Viv sat on the edge, just to be there.

The next day I received a letter from Jude.

Dear Kath:

I was so glad to receive your letter and verses. Yes, they do have you rather snowed, but at least they're trying some different combinations, one of which will bring, or help to bring you out of that fog. I'm sorry your Christmas was so lonely. Naturally, poor timing on top of everything else. The psychiatrist sounds like a fairly decent guy, which makes me breathe a lot easier. I didn't know what to expect from them (in the way of approach, different attitudes, etc.) As each day passes, I hope you become just a little more comfortable, so you can zero in kind of unconsciously on the many thoughts and decisions you are faced with. I realize you can't sit around and ponder on everything; hopefully, your shrink will help you on a couple of issues.

I could go on and on as far as your present and future relationship with Ted—but all the decisions are up to you. It's so difficult not being able to help you at this point, but I can't, as I don't have the answers. You can count on me as support, though, because I truly believe in you and will be behind you 100% on any of your decisions!

I've rambled on long enough. Please take care, and let me hear from you. If I can help in any way, let me know, because I'll be here, Ok?
much love—

Jude

A couple of weeks up north, a few weeks down here in the smog, and I felt strong, somehow. I concluded that if I was to make improvements in my life, I should be doing it in the context of where I lived—with Ted—rather than in a place where I could pretend that nothing had ever happened at home. Intellectually, I understood everything Dr. Rex explained to me about how I was acting out little-girl impulses, and that I needed first to acknowledge that part of me, and accept it, before I could go on. Since that made sense, I was able to gather up all my mental and emotional reserves in an attempt to convince him that I really was getting better. Besides, I'd gotten this far without disaster, so to speak, so couldn't I get through anything?

I guess I convinced him, because he discharged me after three weeks of round two—on the condition that I would immediately seek another therapist when I arrived home. I promised him I would, knowing full well it would be quite unnecessary.

Rebekeh drove me to the airport. While we ate breakfast together, she cried, feeling that I was deserting her; I knew now what it was to be on the other side. It's an accepted fact, though rarely spoken, that when we weep it's for ourselves, and not for those who are gone.

I'd miss her, just as I'd missed Margy, but I had to concentrate on meeting Ted, who was anxious to forget my incarceration. Dwelling on that encounter made leaving the staff less painful, except for Viv and her unconditional acceptance of me. I tried not to think about the inside work I'd avoided. Nothing like arriving emotionally drained—the flight simply wasn't long enough to make up the deficit.

FOURTEEN

Being home again felt like culture shock. I'd been hospitalized for nearly seven weeks, and coming back to everything that had precipitated it was nearly unbearable. Still heavily medicated, I found it difficult to drag myself out of bed; I was lucky to be up by noon. It wasn't at all what I'd expected. Assuming I would be able to function normally as soon as I got home, I hadn't allowed for any emotional lag, and began to wish I'd never left the hospital's warm security.

Jude called and we planned a day of skiing in an attempt to pick up my sagging spirits. This should have been really exciting for me especially since I hadn't skied yet that season, but I was dulled by the meds. I felt extremely fortunate that by midafternoon I hadn't broken anything. We quit early, completely worn out. The genuine joy she'd shown when I drove up that morning lifted my spirits, and I really appreciated her tolerance of a foreign me. In the back of my mind, though, I still felt I wasn't worth the effort.

On Sunday Ted took me to church, and I saw how many people had been praying for me. I felt strange as several congratulated me for being there—the first time since early fall—and for having "gotten through it all." Hurray for Kathy. Then when Heidi saw me, she started crying; I just stood there, feeling like shit.

Kathy, it's just so *good* to see you . . . I can't believe it!

Any Other Song

I didn't think I mattered that much.

Oh, my gosh—but you do! You do! I'm just so happy to see you're Ok! That made me feel again the intense pain that I'd brought to other people, causing so much grief. You certainly made my prayer life more meaningful. *Wow. There I was wanting to help people by offering them something of myself, and ended up being a burden to pray over.*

The whole bout of hospitalizations was like a bad dream, and the reason I was ever admitted was lost to me. The thought of all the anguish I'd withstood threw me into body-racking tears by the time we got home. Ted sadly realized that he wasn't enough to make me feel like a person again; no one would ever be able to satisfy that craving or fill the emptiness that haunted me incessantly. It upset Ted sufficiently to prompt him to take me to a shrink on Monday. That night I was back in the hospital.

> snow's piled up outside
> and inside.
> all my warmth
> has been wrung out
> and stepped on.
>
> i couldn't care less
> if i ever can
> be and do
> what i once was able to.
> it's not enough
> to live for others
> when i don't care about me.
>
> so, where do i go now
> for help
> to become a person again,
> content to live my life
> and give to someone
> without ravaging pain?
> because maybe i do care.
>
> someone, please, show me how.

But there was no one at that reputable private hospital who cared—at all. Ever. The nursing staff was icily professional and remained safely distant; everyone else was nonexistent. Except one man I never understood—one of those people hurt by a lover. I argued with him, until he angrily confronted me with our sameness.

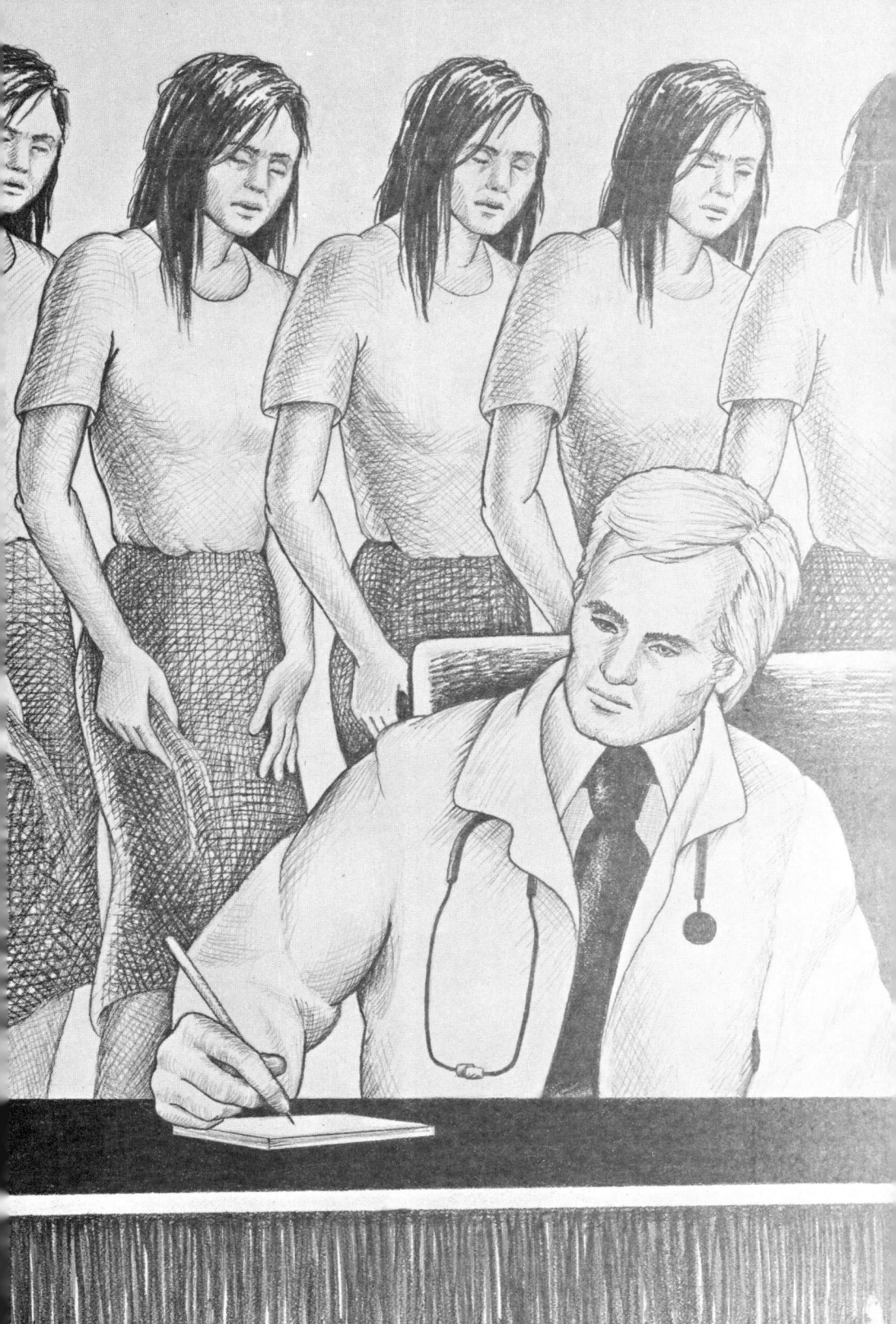

The locked unit was a zoo of adolescents and adults, windowed isolation rooms and narrow little corridors, shabbily carpeted. It operated on behavior mod—you play by their rules, let all of your affect come screaming out, then they'd know that you were working on your problems, and only then would they opt to talk with you, but you had to make the first move. And in every session with my ancient psychiatrist, who looked frighteningly like Captain Ahab from Moby Dick, *he would simply sit there, saying little, obviously out of touch, studying me from miles away.*

Walking back to the unit after a typical session with him, I realized finally that it was all up to me. Only me. No one could help me dig myself out of the pit I was in. My head knew that no one had the patience or stamina to help me. It was frightening to think I might never be undepressed, never find the real me again, and end up locked in there forever. Miriam had warned that it could happen. Wondering where the fighting part of me had gone, the part Mom kept telling me to find and hang on to, I prayed in a last ditch effort to change. Believe with my head, not my heart. And for the first time in a great long while, my mental fog seemed to dissipate.

The next day, things were better inside. I finally understood what Miriam had been saying to me all along, about letting my mind make intelligent decisions instead of letting my emotions run the show. So I saw no reason why I needed to be hospitalized any longer, feeling strong enough to handle anything.

I tested out my decision on Jude when I spent the afternoon with her at home.

Watching you, Kathy, is like seeing a zombie. That's the effect of being drugged. At first I thought you were just nervous about being out of the hospital, but I'd see if you can get your doc to cut off your meds. That's just not you, Kathy, and I don't believe you needed to be in there in the first place!

That was energizing! She helped me believe that it wasn't something I'd forever lost, but that the gnawing depression was accentuated by all the pills. I had sufficient support to announce to the charge nurse Monday morning, as everyone lined up for their goodies, that I was refusing my medication.

I'm sorry, but you can't do that. You'll have to take it up with your doctor first. Take your pills.

No! I'm not going to take them. I don't want them, nor do I need them. I hate the side effects! *That definitely rattled her, as she abruptly turned and stalked back inside the nurses' station.*

Dr. Kran arrived shortly after. Surprisingly, he agreed to keep me off the meds to see how I did. I was practically home free.

Any Other Song

At our session that afternoon, my alertness was increasing, and I felt more like the person I'd always hoped was inside—in control. I was amazed at how coherent I was, and my energy multiplied geometrically. Can't you tell a difference, Dr. Kran?

I agree that there is a noticeable change in you, but there is a quality of unreality to it all.

That's just because you don't know me off the medications! No one here does! Really—this is the best I've felt in six months! Don't you think I'm well enough to go home now? Besides, people who do know me think I don't even belong in here.

Perhaps. But I'd like to see how you do after a few days, first. Your previous doctor had you on the medication for some serious problems he saw in your behavior. I don't want to let you go before you're ready, so that there won't be a repeat performance of your sequential hospitalizations.

But I've taken it all up with the Lord, and I feel quite strong. Wouldn't it be an act of faith in Him on your part if you let me go?

No, I'd call that whistling in the dark. You talked the other doctors into letting you go before you were ready, and here you are. So, I think the best choice is to wait and see how you do off the medication.

That was that. He was frustrating, but I refused to let that dampen my spirits. I went on an all-out campaign to convince the disbelieving staff that I was finished with the fog, by harassing them until they talked to me. They agreed there was a difference but I ignored their reluctance to see it as healthy.

Nance stopped by one evening, asking for insight to help her see what was happening in her life. I was amazed she'd even come to me, and shared with her the exciting prospect I might be discharged on Thursday. I was amazed at all we had weathered together, and intrigued with her assurance that Ted had really changed for the better because of it all. And Tuesday when I was talking with Miriam, she convinced me that the marriage would work out. It had to. I wanted to believe that—with everything in me.

<pre>
          as the dense, steel-gray clouds
           billow threateningly over the
                 too-distant horizon,
                   hazy and blue,
                       i feel
                     trapped.
               my mind never ceases
                    to churn up
                 painful yesterdays
         creating new and vaguely unwanted
</pre>

E. J. Daniel

*solutions to
everpresent problems,
and i want to
run
to that point
when i no longer
hurt.*

*i want
to give
myself
to others in ways
i once knew,
or even to find a
new way,
but the hellish past
has made mutant
my once-familiar talents,
and all i can do is
cry.*

*so, as i vegetate
alone,
i wonder what the
shortest route is
to that
elusive horizon.*

At our Thursday session, Dr. Kran seemed rather secretive. I've been reviewing the social history Ted gave the social worker here, as well as your own medical history. *It must have been eye-opening.* If you don't mind, Kathy, I'd like to talk with Ted before I make any decisions, since he'll be the one responsible for you. *He placed a phone call to Ted right there, while I sat and stared out the window at the barren tree limbs occasionally raking the screen in the chinook wind. The mountains gleamed of spring skiing.*

Kathy, if Ted is willing to take you back, I'll discharge you, but only if you promise to continue seeing me on a regular out-patient basis. I feel there are some really deep problems that need working out, and I'm afraid that sometime one of the impulses that seem to have contributed to your multiple accidents will blow up in your face. *Goodness. How to scare your patient.*

Because I'd put myself into his care and authority, I was obligated to at least consider the possibility that there were some other things that might need correcting. But he seemed to be putting too many pieces into the puzzle, declaring that they fit.

Any Other Song

I'm just afraid for you, Kathy, that once you get out of here, you'll quit coming to see me. *I knew that was true, but for the time being, I played along. If I was going to be considerate of the time invested in me by everyone, I had to continue seeing him—for awhile, anyway. As long as his counseling made sense to me. I owed it to everyone, and most of all to myself. I knew it wasn't going to be easy, and I desperately wished that it could just all be over.*

Going on the premise that Ted had changed, that I had changed—though Lindy sensed I hadn't—I left the circus with Jude to go back, again, however tenuous it felt.

> i write it and
> scream it
> and show it but
> those-in-white don't
> hear can't hear
> won't hear
> me or
> anyone else
> who hurts like hell
> inside . . .
> why?

CONSIDER

1. On Kathy's initial ER visit, what are some of the medical precautions necessary to provide safe care?
2. What were the interferences and obstacles Kathy faced in integrating staff suggestions? What determined the direction she followed?
3. What role does "self-fulfilling prophecy" play in a patient's ability to effect change?
4. What meaningful things in Kathy's life were perceived as lost? What can nursing staff do to ameliorate this sense of grief?
5. What spiritual concerns have/have not been met, and how can these be cared for?

INTERLUDE

Some misty blue and moody Indian summer noon
you came to me
seeking a reason
for why and how
you're where you are.
I listened,
and you talked and cried
and emptied endless tears and bitterness
on me.

After seemingly endless catharsis
I grew frustrated
because you seemed to crave
an answer,
any answer.
But there wasn't one—
not that you would hear.

If there were an instant solution
or a magic pill
I'd gladly give it to you . . .
But there is not.
And when you cried,
it hurt,
Because I can feel, too,
how hard
it really
is.

And I'm sorry . . .

FUGUE

FIFTEEN

One dismal Thursday morning as I scurried to work in the late winter muck, I nearly had an acute anxiety attack. I'd been watching my feet trip along the hallway and in the crosstraffic bumped into Brenda. She didn't seem to recognize me, but her blue scrub dress triggered a grotesque rerun of that unsolicited Thanksgiving, and I fled before she could remember.

> so WHY, Lord
> is there really
> no one
> to cry to
> and share
> my deepest fears with?
>
> WHY
> am i
> alone
> in my tears
> and persistent pain?

I guess everyone knew all along that it wouldn't work. I wanted so badly to believe that Ted had really changed, and I thought I'd even sensed a difference in him when we took a spring ski vaca-

Any Other Song

tion the weekend before he started his surgery rotation—the killer. But in the middle of the sunny snow, inside, I heard something else. So I wasn't surprised when Ted, after one month together, became again everything that I remembered him being six months and more before. Of course, I felt it was all him, even though Lindy's accusation that I hadn't changed, either, echoed hauntingly in my mind. I'd been through enough forced personality alterations though, to shut out what I didn't want to hear, and proceeded to show everyone that Kathy was all better.

Three short weeks into the quarter, I noticed Ted wasn't aware of his reverted behavior, nor my half-hearted attempts to convey to him that I wasn't happy with the old Ted. On advice force-fed during my therapeutic hospitalizations, I decided to speak out—loudly.

Look, Ted! Everyone said you'd changed. I wanted to believe them, but you haven't changed at all. You've put us right back where we were six months ago! What does it take?

Oh, Kathy—I've changed, really. I just got caught up again in school. I forgot. I'm sorry.

Shit! You give me that line every time! I'm just not in the same place emotionally as I was before, and I refuse to bite. Really—this time I'll leave. *There—I'd said it, but there were no cheers.*

He stood there stunned, his ski-tanned face slowly paling as he withdrew into his customary silence. I was a little amazed I'd actually hit him with that. I'd been feeling so powerful lately, that I'd even terminated with Dr. Kran.

My track record with shrinks was nothing to brag about, but when they began suggesting options I couldn't accept, I stopped going. Dr. Kran insisted on leaving open the option of separation, which didn't make sense to me if I was supposed to be considerate of others' feelings, even though Miriam said she, too, would rather see us separate awhile than to watch me disintegrate. But what upset me most about Kran was that on our third outpatient session, he commented that he was beginning to get to like me. How heartwarming. After two more sessions with him, me getting nowhere, I called in and cancelled my next appointment. That was the week before Ted and I went skiing, when it appeared that things had improved in the marriage; we'd be out of town anyway, and I just felt I didn't need to be talking to a shrink. Then he went on vacation, so that eliminated several weeks.

I was at work one afternoon when Dr. Kran called to find out what had happened to me. Unready for him, I went to pieces in-

side, vaguely agreeing because of his persistence, to come in again the following week. But after I'd mulled it over a short while, I changed my mind and wrote him a letter of termination, bluntly writing what I couldn't say. His reply made me feel guilty as hell.

> Dear Kathy:
> Your letter arrived yesterday and left me saddened, especially since you didn't keep your appointment this morning. I was saddened because I see you, through the letter, as being terribly perplexed yet, and badly needing someone to confide in. There are so many elements in your letter which you need to elaborate on that I sincerely wish you would come in and discuss them with me. I really would like to continue working with you and feel badly about your wanting to terminate.
> I have 11:00 AM Friday open now, and will hold that time for you. I urge you to come in then so we can elaborate on these issues. I do miss working with you since, as I said, "I do like you."

That letter reminded me of the time in my advanced English class in high school when I contested a low grade on a paper I hadn't really worked on, and ended up receiving an apology from the teacher, plus a higher grade. I didn't deserve it, and knew how very difficult it was for her to admit to hastiness in grading. She wasn't that kind of teacher. Neither was Dr. Kran an apologetic physician. But it was too late for me to change my mind. That would have been out of character.

I spent a lot of time with Jude, leaning heavily on her for the support I was too afraid to seek from Jo or Lindy. Sensing a pending earthquake, Jude suggested that I consult another psychiatrist. I was forcing her to her breaking point.

I wasted two weeks trying to get an initial appointment with any one of the psychiatrists Jude referred me to, but no one could see me sooner than a month. That made me feel like shit. Easter was staring me in the face, and I had unwittingly put another pressure on myself by agreeing to give my incredible testimony during the special morning services. I couldn't see how anyone would believe the Lord was working, or had ever worked in my life, after hearing all that had happened. It seemed everyone expected the ghastly trauma to be over at long last, and that I was on the way out and up—but it didn't feel that way to me. I had tried to use all the resources available to me, but I just wasn't able to put into practice what I heard, and no one could understand that.

Because of the intense pressure I couldn't get out from under, my

Any Other Song

body collapsed on Monday. It forced me to admit that everything was not alright. There just weren't any other explanations for why I was physically ill. When I failed to improve, unable to eat or keep anything down, it was time to see Dr. Reilley.

I made an appointment to see him in his office rather than in clinic so I could explain my weight loss. I didn't need to be examined for something so blatantly psychosomatic. But he took me over to a booth in the ER anyway. After a cursory exam, he left me lying on the stretcher. In a few minutes he returned with a Family Practice resident.

Kathy, this is Dr. Cook. He's on call for Emergency Psychiatry. *My nausea suddenly returned.*

Now, Kathy only comes to see me in a crisis. She's an old friend of mine, so take good care of her. *He smiled gently at me.* I'll see you later, Kathy. *And he left.*

In a slight state of shock I followed the resident back to the very same room in which I'd sat six months earlier with Dr. Westberg. I was now facing something I felt would never *be necessary again. At 4:00 that Thursday afternoon, I began to wish I was someone else, somewhere other than where I was.*

So what's bothering you? *So how's the stock market? I wasn't in the mood to talk with this jerk, until I remembered that if I wanted help, I had to talk. I hesitated, but there seemed to be no other way out.* Are you suicidal right now? *Sigh.*

Not exactly. I mean, I don't have any plan made or anything. But, if on walking out of this hospital, a truck happened to unite me with the pavement, I couldn't care less.

Well, I think that's enough of a reason to hospitalize you.

Wrong! I'm not going back into the hospital! Not this one. Not any one! Now now. I don't need that.

Where's your husband right now?

Ted's not interested in where I am.

I want to talk to him. Is he at home? *I nodded, and he left to drop the bombshell. Terrified, I telephoned Jude. She was aghast.*

Kathy! You don't need another hospitalization, unless I'm really not reading you correctly. Just push to get an outpatient therapist and get out of there. You've already seen that hospitalization doesn't work for you.

Jude, I've been trying to get hold of those docs, but no one can see me for at least 3 weeks! *And I sat there, alone. There was nothing else to say.*

Ted walked into the room at that point, with the resident behind him. That was quick. Ted made it very clear that he was violently opposed to another hospitalization. The shrink got involved with that declaration. When the assembled group of minds couldn't agree, they left Ted and me alone while someone tried to contact one of the private psychiatrists Jude had mentioned. Ted continued to stare unbelievingly at me, as I stood propped up against the wall, studying the floor, hiding behind my hair, arms folded protectively.

What's happened, Kathy? *I still wasn't in the mood for talking, especially to him. I turned to stare coldly at him, unamazed anymore that he hadn't seen it all coming, couldn't understand, and never would. He couldn't have prevented it, anyway. It was too late.*

> it's all me.
> only me. just
> me.
> no one else
> making decisions,
> giving me a reason to
> go on,
> helping me to see me as i am
> or as i appear to be, maybe
> accepting myself.
> only me.

The shrink, the resident, and a psychiatric social worker came back in en masse after a long icy silence. Remaining withdrawn against the chipped plaster wall, I felt I was crumbling apart.

We were able to talk with Dr. Bortolli, and she's willing to see you on an outpatient basis, but doesn't have an opening for several weeks.

I know that! But I don't think I can last that long.

Well, that's why Ms Fritz is here. She's agreed to see you in the interim, if that's alright with you.

Everyone was watching me, waiting; when she finally smiled at me, I nodded. Nothing to lose.

I have an opening tomorrow morning at 9:00. Is that a good time for you? *I shrugged.* Do you think you'll be Ok til then? *She seemed concerned, slowly dissolving all my negative stereotypes of social workers.*

I didn't think I'd be alright, but I nodded anyway, extremely anx-

Any Other Song

ious to fly out of there. It was 7:00 when the little group broke up in an uneasily settled conclusion. To me, it was merely another band-aid, an intellectual stop-gap.

> Consultation note: 24-year-old female was referred by Dr. Reilley for evaluation. She is the wife of a 3rd year med student. The couple was married for 4 years with good relationship until he was required to be away from home a lot, which initiated a series of hospitalizations including here, after an OD during therapy with Dr. Westberg, followed by another hospitalization at which time she re-entered the marital relationship. Finding it very similar, she again required hospitalization surrounding suicide ideation and entered into another therapeutic relationship with Dr. Kran, which terminated several weeks ago. She feels very depressed and with suicidal ideation at present partially surrounding being unable to find another therapist and partially secondary to a recent argument with husband and possible separation.
>
> Mental status is within normal limits; no loose associations. Affect is depressed. Impression: situation anxiety and depression. Kay Fritz will see the patient in the morning. Patient is willing to go home with husband, and if not working out, will stay with friend or return here before attempting suicide.

Friday morning I was apprehensive about seeing this new counselor whose office was right across the hall from Dr. Westberg's. I dreaded running into him, feeling as though I should apologize to him because things hadn't worked out. As I was hesitating, Ms Fritz invited me into her office. She seemed liberated, around thirty, and open, which helped me decide to trust her. She didn't sit clear on the opposite side of the room, as Westberg had, and honestly seemed to care about me. I had to talk to someone, or I was going to explode.

You know, Kathy, I don't usually just pick up clients like this.

Why did you do it?

You seemed a more interesting case than the usual long-term neurotics that walk into the ER. *Blunt. But honest. And talking with her gradually helped calm me down. I found myself opening up to her in ways I'd been afraid to before with anyone for fear of being rehospitalized, which I continued to tell myself would never again be necessary.*

I patched my way through the weekend, and met with her again on Monday. She put me back on the Stelazine to quell the apprehension that refused to dissipate, being careful to only give me enough until we met again on Friday. That really angered me, because she was depriving me of an option. But it also felt very good knowing that I was being taken seriously for once. Finally, very seriously.

Ted was outraged that I was back on medication, so after a while, I quit taking the pills—partly to please him, partly because I denied that I needed them. I had a bad habit of being oddly selective about which areas I would be obedient in. Ms Fritz, however, wasn't too pleased with the move. That prompted a rather lengthy discussion about doing what I wanted and needed, as opposed to what others wanted, and who ultimately was most important. Logically, I was supposed to matter the most, and I intellectually understood that, but I couldn't accept it. It had always been everyone else first, then me.

Friday faded into Monday, which hurried too quickly into another Friday. For some forgotten reason, I quit taking the Stelazine again, and was strung out when I met with Ms Fritz again Friday morning.

Don't the pills help, Kathy?

I suppose they do.

Then why don't you take them?

I don't know.

She sighed, studying me for awhile. Well, I want you to take one now, and then come back this afternoon at 3:00. The Stelazine should have helped your anxiety by then.

My insides were screaming, I was so tense, so I took two pills. I had a casual lunch with Ted as though nothing was going on, and not surprisingly, he was oblivious to my raging state of mind. We even had a drink together, celebrating our first lunch out with each other in too long. But I didn't feel like confiding in him. Back at work, because of the accelerating churning, I took several more pills before going back to see Ms Fritz that afternoon. I wanted to stop feeling anything.

Kathy, have you been drinking?

What a slam. I hadn't thought my stupor would be so obvious. Uh, it's the Stelazine.

Dead silence. I wanted to run. How many? I only told you to take one.

I'm sorry. Really! But I was just too strung out, and when the two pills this morning didn't help slow me down, I took a couple more. *Tears welled up, dripping on my tense, clammy hands. My head was pounding. I'd really blown it.*

Is your mouth dry? *I slowly nodded, surprised that she would*

Any Other Song

know. Well, after seeing you this morning, I put a bed on hold for you. I rarely hospitalize patients, especially just before the weekend. But we've tried over the last couple of weeks to work things out, and it hasn't been successful. So, I'd like you to walk with me over to the hospital so I can get you admitted. Ok?

>   bittersweet moments
>   of any past and pungent summer
>   whisper
>   as i lay
>   face up, caressed gently in
>   foot-high reedy grass
>   between hedgerows of lilac
>   bordering Fountain Creek,
>   the full moon playing
>   hide-and-seek
>   with pale clouds drifting across
>   the star-filled sky.
>
>   Oh, God, it was
>   so good then,
>   as hoot owls
>   conversed sparingly with
>   late-night pigeons.
>   soft was each dream
>   soothing every thought
>   of secret fantasies.
>
>   Jesus, what happened to
>   those tomorrows?

A distant Kathy strolled reluctantly across the courtyard with Ms Fritz, over to the Emergency Psychiatry Department. Upon arrival, as she busied herself with the admission forms, I excused myself to get some personal things I'd purposefully forgotten in the lab. Once up there, I immediately called Jude, but no one was home. Stopping by work to see if I'd like to take a coffee break with her, Annie waited until my tears were controlled sufficiently to explain to her where I was supposed to be.

Why don't you call them up and ask if it's alright for you to just stay with us for the weekend, if it's a matter of you being alone. Ok? Call and ask!

I was hesitant to accept her offer, preferring instead to just run. But I called downstairs anyway.

Kathy! Where are you now? *Ms Fritz was losing her patience.*

At work.

Why don't you just get your things, and come down—*now. Her tone was even and insistent, and I left Annie in tearful resignation.*

When I finally re-appeared downstairs, Ms Fritz was silent. My second thoughts about it wanted to surface. Would it be alright if I went home first to get my clothes?

She dropped her pen on the desk and just stared at me incredulously. You know, you complain about not being heard, and not being taken seriously, but when you are, you honestly expect me to let you go? I don't think so. Dr. Melk is waiting for us upstairs, and I have a 4:00 appointment. Let's go, Kathy.

She took my arm, escorting me up to the eighth floor. And the very thing I said would never happen to me ever again was happening.

> Admit note: 25-year-old female, wife of medical student, has 3 past psych hospitalizations including here last fall. I've seen her twice a week the past 2 weeks while she's been waiting for an appointment with Dr. Bortolli. Crux of therapy has been looking at options patient has besides becoming self-destructive. She feels no one really takes her seriously. Patient feels husband thinks she can shape up if she decides to do so, and is manipulating people, he feels. I believe this is a change for her to tell the therapist she can't hang on before attempting suicide.
>
> Last night she talked to husband regarding a separation. He said no deal. Patient feels at dead end. She was able to stop herself from OD, doesn't think she can get through the day, or even wants to. She took six 2mg Stelazine since 11 AM to "calm down."
>
> Mental status—oriented X3, depressed affect, ambivalent, needs and asks for structure. No thought disorder. Confused, inconsistent thinking. Impression—borderline marital maladjustment. Admit to 8 East; hook up with long-term therapist.

SIXTEEN

*this time
those-in-white-in-colors
seem on my side,
caring about me—
but my friends don't,
saying I'm manipulative
and can be/do
all that I'm supposed to be/do
regardless
of how I'm feeling.*

*and I think I'll just run—
find anyone
who meets me where I am
not where they say I should be—
lovingly, gently helping
me accept that point,
so I can grow into
a better me—
somehow.*

I was flat and despondent from the pills I'd ingested when I called Ted around dinnertime to ask him to bring me some clothes. There was a long silence.
    Ted. I'm on 8 East.

Any Other Song

What are you doing up there?

I've been admitted! So can you find time to bring me some clothes? *An hour later he showed up, sullen and distant. Where was the love?*

I suppose you'll call again when you want to see me. And limit my visits to you, like before.

No, Ted. You can come by tomorrow.

Gee, thanks. *And stalked out. Big deal.*

As I sat in my darkening room, I could think of no reason to try and keep on anymore, since the option I chose upon getting out of the hospital before—to make my marriage work—had just failed. So, this time around, I vowed to succeed at what I was afraid of last time I was there.

> lonely
> in a steel cage
> lonely
> in a solo room
> me and no one
> looking for answers
> refusing to be found
> on an endless night
> of ghoulish dreams
> that never
> should have started . . .

Saturday afternoon, Ted did come by; we again failed to communicate, even civilly. I stormed out of my room and down the hall toward the door to see him out, while he followed vainly behind. He left in tears. The rest of the day I sulked, wishing that the last time we'd gone skiing I'd been able to do what I'd planned. Careening down the slope, out of control from too many pills, I'd aimed for the trees at the edge of the run, but the deep powder cushioned my collision with the tree trunk. Ted was mortified when he found me buried in the snow, wrapped snugly around the tree; I was numb.

I sat in my room waiting for nightfall, when everyone else would be down in the dayroom watching the tube. I rigged a noose from part of a sheet and hung it from the bathroom door. I wasn't even thinking or feeling when I put it around my neck and slowly let it tighten from the weight of my body. But it didn't happen as fast as I'd hoped, and just when I feared every vessel in my head would explode from the pressure, I chickened out and fumbled frantically at the sheet to loosen the strangling noose. I just stood there in the dark, the taut sheet in my limp hands, wondering what the heck I was doing.

What's going on Kathy? *One of the nurses had strolled down the hall and wandered into my room. She watched me hand her the sheet, a strained look on her face as she untied the knots.* You know this won't solve anything. *Staring at the floor, I nodded.* Let's talk about it. Come on out in the hall. *I followed short, weathered Addy out of the room and waited as she disposed of the sheet; I avoided any eye contact.*

Would it help at all to have a third person in on your conversations with your husband? Because we can certainly do that, especially if it'll prevent things like this from happening. You should've come and talked with one of us after he left, rather than go and vegetate alone in your room. You know? *I probably needed to hear her cold, hard logic, but I preferred empathy; not finding it there, I withdrew further.*

I don't want you alone in your room any more tonight, so go on out to the dayroom with everyone else that's still up. When you're ready to go to bed, then you can have your sleeper. Does that make sense?

Again I nodded as I slowly stumbled away, distant and pensive.

Sunday I watched enviously as other doctors came in and visited their patients, but Ms Fritz, who'd said she'd put me in there so she wouldn't worry all weekend about me, wasn't around. And the last thing I wanted was to bother anyone. So I went in to sit in the orange dayroom and write off the afternoon.

Apparently having gotten the news from Ted, Jo and Ron stopped by. I let them know that I was considering a trial separation to put myself back together again first, because the marriage wasn't working in its present context. But Jo precisely and pointedly disagreed with my logic.

You *know* that's not scriptural, Kathy! I think God wants you to be married to Ted, and He wants you to learn how to love him—which you haven't been doing for a *long* time. I believe you can work it out, if you want to; but if you still feel that separation is the answer, then, because I love you as a sister, I have to tell you that I see that move as blatantly disobedient to God's Word. I just have to tell you that. *That sounded pretty consistent with Ted.*

I don't know what kind of response she expected from me after that blast, but it certainly blew me away. Maybe Ron sensed that, because he didn't add anything, but gently encouraged me to keep trying. They left not soon enough, and I slumped over the table in emotional shock. Two of the staff had overheard the conversation,

Any Other Song

and interrupted my empty reasonings. The burly, bearded ex-football jock hurried out to intercept Jo and Ron before they left the ward; Braye sat down gently beside me.

Kathy, you don't have to take that kind of talk—not from anyone. What's important is *you*, and what you think is best. *She knew that what she was saying was relevant; an ex-nun would understand where my feelings of guilt and responsibility were coming from.* You've got to stop letting other people lay their trips on you, and get you down. You're the one who's got to live with yourself and your decisions—not anyone else. No one can make those decisions for you, either. *Greg came back and sat down with us.* Next time, come and get one of us to sit in on your visits. Can you do that? *I really wanted to believe her.*

We want to help, Kathy, but you've got to let us in.

Their support and concern was welcome, but I realized it just wasn't enough to keep me going. I grew more silent and distant. Sensing my frustration, they dragged me down the hall to toss the medicine ball for awhile, rather than leave me to stew.

Greg heaved the monstrous ball at me over and over, trying to hurt me enough to elicit anger that I could take out on him. Come on, Kathy! You're not really trying. Hit me right here! You can't hurt me.

Come on and get it out, Kathy!

Greg and Braye had me in the middle, and a couple of times I got mad enough to hurl the ball at him, particularly when he jammed my thumb. But after several grinding minutes I just dropped it, because I couldn't see through my tears. I can't get mad at you two—you care too much. I'm afraid I'll hurt you.

You're not going to hurt us, Kathy.

I just feel like lying down for awhile.

You'll be Ok? *Sure, Braye. It'd be no great loss, anyway.*

You come out and get one of us if you start feeling bad, alright? *Yes, Greg. But it's not worth the bother.*

Collapsing on my bed, I buried my head in the pillow to muffle the deep sobbing. I felt like I was being pulled in half—do this, no don't, what about that?, be the person you know you should, we know you can do it—on and on, ad infinitum. I cried even harder because I knew that I was expected to do it alone, and I just couldn't. God was asking too much of me.

The tears ran out I was so tired, and then part of me found a way out. I wanted to run, but watched in disbelief as the nightgown was pulled out. I lay back down, tied it snugly around my neck, head under my pillow. *But fear again overwhelmed me, and I clawed at the suffocating mass to undo what I must not have really wanted to do. I jumped up, head pounding, and stared out the Plexiglas windows at all of the green trees and summer grass; seeing the absurdity of what I'd been attempting to do. That just wasn't me.*

Monday morning I sat through another goals meeting with all of the patients and staff on a different team than when I was hospitalized before. Afterward, the head nurse approached me; what I'd managed to mumble I'd forgotten, *and couldn't figure out what I'd said wrong.*

Kathy, since this is a repeat hospitalization for you, we have a policy of having the team meet individually with such patients so that we can better understand what we as staff can do to help.

Nice to know they agreed I was a mistake. With everyone?

It's only to give you a chance to tell us what your expectations are of us.

I'm not going to get grilled?

There may be some questions, but only for clarification. Ok? Someone will be out to bring you in; oh, give us fifteen minutes. *She walked primly off to join the already gathered Orange team. It sounded really fun, but I forgot it ever happened. It wasn't worth their effort.*

Later in the day I met with Ms Fritz and Dr. Melk, and told them, embarrassed, of my attempts.

Why didn't you call me—or get one of the staff?

I didn't know you were reachable. I didn't want to be a bother. *She looked at me, shaking her head.*

This was going to be a relatively short hospitalization for you this time. We'd been thinking about discharge for tomorrow or so, but I don't know now. *I sat staring at the floor, terrified at the prospect of being turned loose.* How about if I come up later today and talk with you again?

If that's Ok?

I will if you want me to, Kathy. *She was trying to get me to say what I really wanted.*

Then please, do. *I wondered why it was so impossible during all of my other hospitalizations to be honest, but it always felt like I was being too demanding. I really wasn't worth the trouble, you know.*

Early in the afternoon the Associate Pastor of our church came by to converse with what was left of me, sharing his disappointment over my partial decision to leave Ted, and I prayed he would

Any Other Song

leave before I fell totally apart in front of his gentle concern. I just wasn't able to make anyone happy anymore. What kind of raunchy person was I to dump on whomever I saw? Let's just stop right here. Leave me alone, and forget I ever lived. Ok?

The staff said the pressure came from my friends, but they seemed unaware that they were pressuring me from the other direction. But Sable had spent some thoughtful time with me.

Why do you suppose you got married when you did, Kathy? *That's a good one.* What's happened to change your feelings?

It probably sounds immature, but, I had dreams of going to faraway places and saw Ted as the door. But instead of growing magically closer or doing free things together, he traded me in for medical school . . . I guess that was the start of it. Too bad Sable wasn't around more to talk to so I could figure things out better.

And for some reason, I watched as slow incisions appeared in parallel rows up my forearm, making the hurt inside less intense, externalizing the pain. But when I met with Ms Fritz a couple of hours later, what I'd done visibly upset her. She looked intently at me, in me, through me, tears streaming down my face.

That's not the best way to tell me you're not ready to go home. *I looked down at my carved-up arms, hair falling down to hide it, and slowly shook my head. Why were those cuts there? What was going on?*

How do you feel right now?

I hesitated, horribly ashamed, choking from the lump in my throat, but forced myself to think about what was racing in my crazy head. I keep dwelling on slipping down to the lab and ripping off some blank scripts so I can just get it over with.

She let out a deep, slow sigh. Not only could that get you into a lot of trouble because it's illegal, but it's not a good idea. I don't want you to have the chance, so give me the key to the lab. *I was beginning to resent my freedom being taken away, but concluded that was her way of showing me she cared. I really did want to trust her. She was offering me an alternative, and I stared at her outstretched, open hand, wanting to feel her concern, but wanting also to run. I gave her the key.*

Thank you.

We exchanged penetrating looks, deadly serious, before she stood up to leave. I was so angry and disgusted with myself I thought I'd explode. I hurried back to my room. Unnoticed and alone, I sat huddled on the cold floor in a corner of the darkened

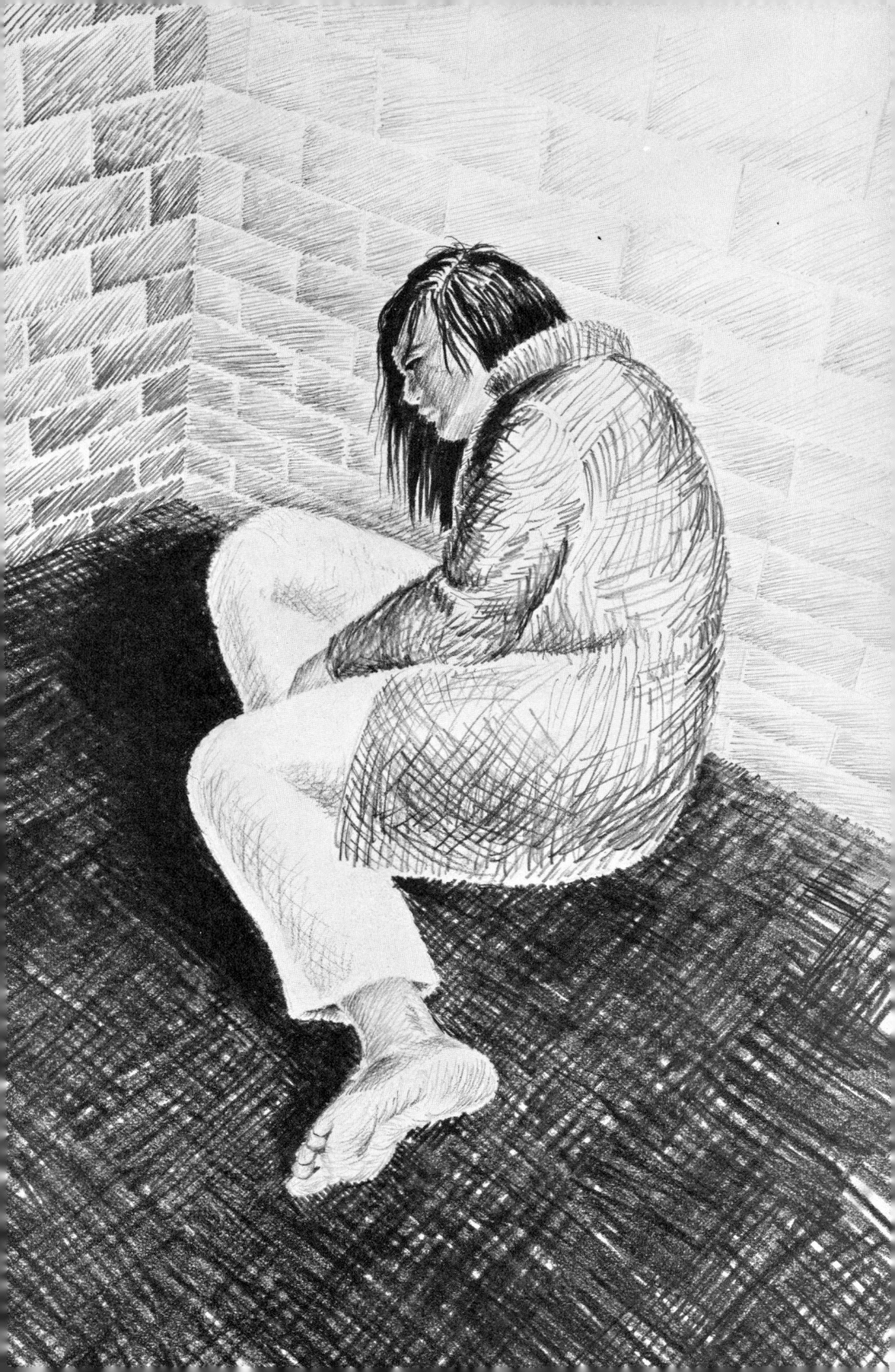

bathroom, rocking gently until I felt my brains smashing against the tiled wall, and as tears mingled with the blood in my convulsing sobbing. Stupid, stupid! I couldn't take it anymore! God, please just let me go! Oh, God . . . please . . .

In small group the next day, I made myself verbalize what I was feeling—that I wasn't ready to be discharged. Dr. Melk understood, but those-in-white gave me privileges, which didn't make sense as I was still feeling too destructive.

Kathy, it's your responsibility to seek out a staff person when you're feeling down, rather than expect us to read you.

As I wandered back to my room, I saw Cory, who'd cared about me so long before.

Kathy! It's so good to see you! *She hugged me warmly.*

Here? *I was surprised.*

Better here than dead. *The heart of the matter.*

Sure, but I feel like a failure to be up here again.

It's always better to get help than to run, you know.

But, Cory, it's too hard! It doesn't work that way!

But we're here. *She smiled warmly.*

But I'm on the wrong side . . . *I heard her concern, savoring it, like a sponge sopping up whatever support I could. I turned to leave, disappointed she was on the other team and wasn't free to talk with me. She was the only nurse left that mattered. Everyone else was oblivious to me, and continued to urge me to make a decision and stick to it, but soon!*

One warm afternoon I just left the ward for awhile, wanting to see how hard it was to just take off. No one saw me sneak out the locked door behind one of the docs, and I flew down the stairs and out into the sunshine. My agitation had accelerated, but once free of the mecca, the flailing slowed. It was too bright outside; it didn't fit. Life was apparently still carrying on, people functioning as though nothing was wrong, as though everything had always worked. I felt strangely detached—a figment of my own imagination.

When I found myself outside the apartment, I hesitated before going in, momentarily undecided. I beelined for the bathroom, but Ted had hidden what I was looking for. In a rage I stormed through the house, ripping open drawers and cabinets until I found the pills. See! No one could stop me. Not Ted, not the staff—not even God! And I cried.

On the back porch, I finished off the left-over liquor, hating the cheery chirping birds, the sickening summer sunshine. It should

Any Other Song

have been cloudy, pouring down freezing rain. *Then I panicked—what if I hadn't taken enough? What if all this did was knock me out? What if Ted came home and found me, and it wasn't too late? Then he'd really hate me. Everyone would!*

Suddenly it was all too confusing. I jumped up, knowing I had to leave, but needing to find out if I'd swallowed enough or not. Somewhere between here and there, I found a phone, and called some emergency room. Oddly, the nurse answering sounded unusually concerned, urging me to come in. I just laughed.

Do you have any transportation, or can you call a friend to help?

Then the tears came, as there was no one left to call. Just forget it. Ok? I'm only another crazy on a psych ward. *And hung up.*

I found myself standing outside the heavy door to the floor, trying to rationalize that it would serve them right when they found me passed out in my room. The door suddenly swung open before I was ready.

Where've you been, Kathy? *Ike was rather intimidating, but I glowered at his big black hulk as I stalked past, veering toward my room before I collapsed.* Kathy. We received a call, and I think you need to come with me down to the Emergency Room.

I whirled around defiantly. What!?

Sit down in this wheelchair. We're going downstairs.

Screw you! You're not taking me anywhere!

Ike stood his ground. Don't fight me, Kathy. Because I care, I'm taking you down there. So, come on. *If I fought, it would make everything worse than it already was. What a sight, to be dragged down to the ER in restraints. Everyone would know I was really crazy, then. And I hated myself more for having even gone back to the ward. I withdrew inside, fading passively away so the humiliation and pain of being pumped out another time wouldn't seem to matter as much. But I'll always remember their faces as I was brought in for treatment. I'd rather die...*

The midget bitch of a charge nurse marched into the same old cubicle, clanging the same equipment, a sneer on her fiery face.

Well, you know what's next. This was a stupid shit thing to do to yourself! Stick your arm over so I can get a line in you. *Ike's gargantuan frame blended into the wall as I faded into oblivion.*

It was dark inside when I woke up. The normal deafening din of the ER had subsided, the lights half on. One-in-white sat next to the stretcher.

Hi, Kath. How're you feeling?

Amy! *I was so surprised to see her. We'd worked with each other*

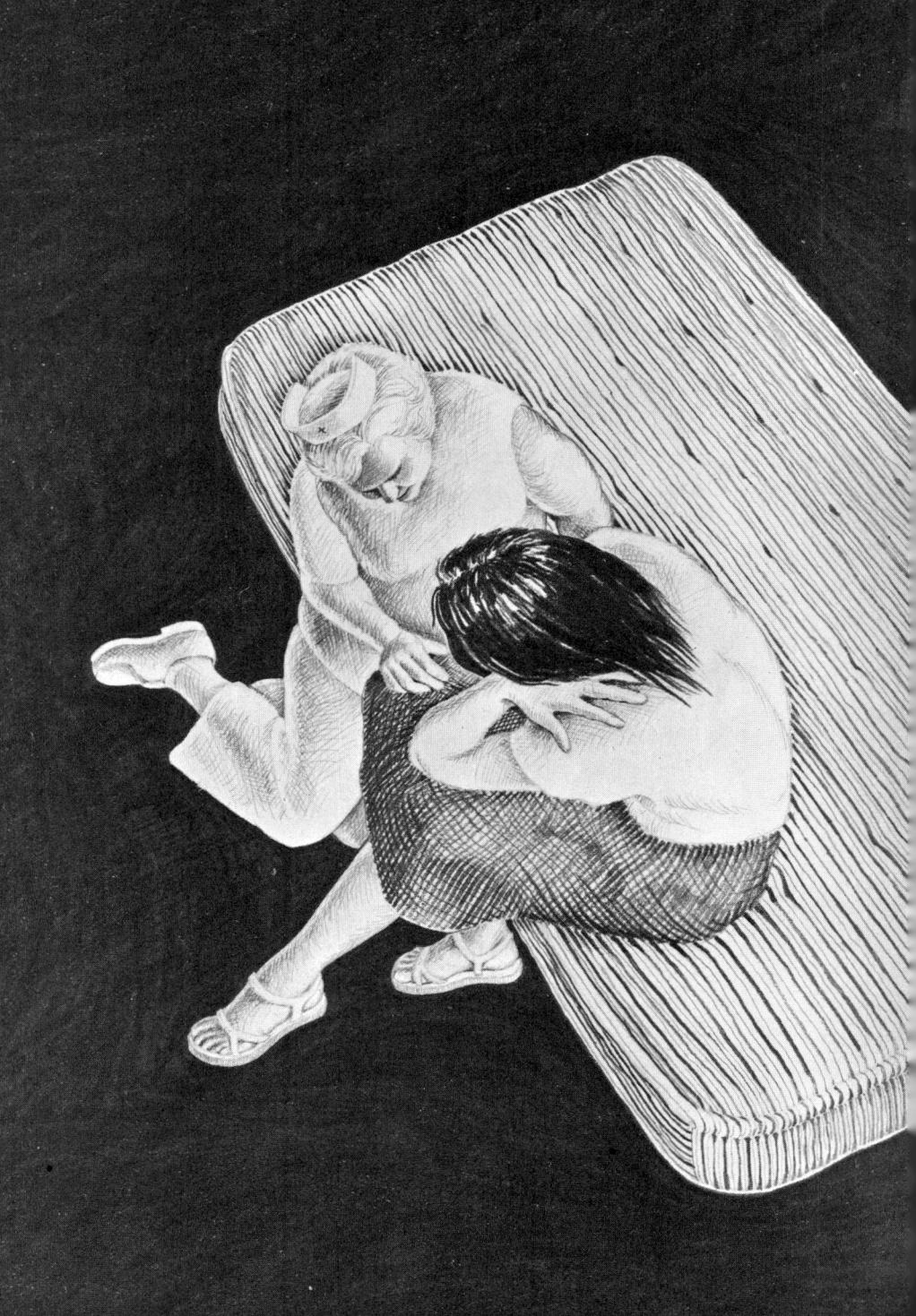

for awhile not so long ago, but she'd transferred to another department. What a way to run into her. What time is it?

Three AM. Since we weren't busy tonight, Julie and I kept you here, rather than farming you up to Intensive. *She squeezed my hand, her big warmth softening the pain, as I grogged back out of touch.*

When I woke up later, Amy was gone, but, out of the nightmare came Cory, waiting to take me back.

Ready, Kathy?

Cory, this isn't going to work! Don't you see? I just can't go back! I don't want to be here. This wasn't supposed to turn out like this at all! I've been crazy too long to be able to get away from not coping. Please, just let me leave!

She looked at me, saddened, and I broke down. Nothing more was said as she wheeled me through the ER, past the blue staff, my head buried. I felt like a piece of defective merchandise being returned for repair, under the delusion I could be fixed. Inside I was primed for an explosion—all the stops had finally been pulled, and nothing was going to stop me, because nothing could.

Upstairs the staff was unusually cautious, and I found myself stripped and locked into seclusion. As if that could calm the raging storm inside! As if I needed to be alone! I sat huddled in the blankets on the mattress in a corner of the icy gray box, wracked with tears, clutching, trying to hold myself together, because I knew if I let go, if I let that anger out, I'd fall apart, and never ever get out of there. But the isolation was too great, my head too confused, my controls burnt out. The mushrooming panic was interrupted hours later when the door was unlocked. In the open doorway stood Julie.

I'll just be a little while, thanks. *She stepped inside, sitting softly beside me on the edge of the blue-striped mattress.* Hi, Kathy. I just wanted to see how you were doing. *Understanding. Accepting.*

Then I broke into sobs. I was so ashamed to have her see me like that. Why, why God, didn't You just let me die! *I couldn't begin to feel the empathy I know was there. After squeezing my arm to say what couldn't be said, she took her warmth, her sanity, and left, the closing door booming shut inside, alone. Alone.*

> and i wonder why
> it has to hurt
> so deeply
> that i won't ever forget—
> not on any gray rainy afternoon
> misty blue and lonely, my self
> apart under a

Any Other Song

> *drizzling over-summered oak.*
> *and there's no one there*
> *to hold my clammy hand*
> *to warm away the dread*
> *and understand*
> *and care.*
>
> *and i wonder when*
> *or if*
> *it will ever*
> *ever*
> *end?*

One afternoon I sat making a token effort at a clay pot, mostly poking holes in the walls that weren't strong enough, in rhythm to the pounding of leather tooling. The lethargy was depressing.

Hey, you! What are you making? *I looked up from my puttering.*

Oh, Annie! *Ashamed for her to see me there, I almost turned her away.* Feeling just super being so productive!

Come on, Kath. It's Ok. It's not forever . . .

And days followed days, broken sporadically by undeserved gestures: a plant from Darley, visits with Annie, hugs from Nance. But it wasn't enough. I needed too much, and no one could humanly commit themselves to that degree of need. I was standing in the corner of the day room when Greg suddenly shook me by the shoulders.

Hey, Kathy! What did you do here? *He raised my hand, turning it over, and I noticed the blood dribbling steadily onto the carpet. I wondered why my arm was partially dissected; it wasn't hurting.* Let's go clean you up. *He guided me into the nurses' station, past gawking faces. That I didn't remember getting cut wasn't surprising, for I'd accepted the fact that I'd always be the way I was—out of touch, distant, and useless.*

Several weeks later Jude picked me up at the hospital to help me do what I never thought I could or would—get an apartment of my own. As we were browsing through one complex, she chanced to see my forearm and looked at me in disgust.

Don't let the manager see that! *She echoed well what I felt for myself.*

I put the money down for the apartment, arranged for the movers to get it over with in a day, and transferred to a new department at work. If that, plus my own car, didn't change the direction I'd been going in I didn't know what would.

Dr. Melk said that he wanted me to spend one night there alone, on pass, in my new apartment, to get used to the way things were going to feel when I was discharged. I spent the day getting moved in, unboxing, arranging; the phone was even installed. But by evening I'd had enough, and fled back to the hospital. My bed there would miss me, you know. Dr. Melk had said I could even call the ward if I felt bad, and maybe show up in the middle of the night if necessary. But the thought of attempting to occupy myself for part of the evening was terrifying, so I opted to suffer the consequences of his disappointment in my failure rather than endure what I couldn't.

I'd moved myself and all of my belongings out of Ted's life just like that. In one day, while he'd been on call. So I wouldn't have time to react to my second thoughts about moving out. Rationally, I'd proved beyond a doubt that I couldn't survive with Ted at home, but—could I do it alone? That evening, back on the ward, I braced as Ted roared onto the floor, nearly in tears.

Well, you finally did it! You hate me *that* much, don't you, to strip me of everything in the house! At least I know it's all over.

At first I thought he was going to punch me out, but he took off as soon as he'd vented his anger. Fine. It was one more confirmation that I was a truly worthless person to hurt someone that much.

And I no longer knew myself. My Christian friends and husband no longer knew me. All those-in-white said I could make it—anyway. They said I deserved much more than what I'd had. Numbly, I asked the Lord for help, but He didn't answer. And it was just me, straddling the chasm between those who knew Him and those who didn't, wanting acceptance from both, finding support from neither.

Termination from the hospital commenced the day after the moving weekend, and I braced for the plunge into separateness, knowing I wasn't ready, thinking I might make it, plodding on for lack of any other direction to take. I wanted to continue seeing Ms Fritz, but professionalism made that impossible, because the next day I was to begin seeing my long-awaited outpatient therapist. The weeks shared with Ms Fritz were gone, and I was torn that our time together was over. She knew me, and I trusted her, but it was finished. The contrast between my discharge this time and the December nightmare was astounding—I wasn't so angry at the staff; it hurt deeper.

irony
when in spring
instead of

Any Other Song

     budding green
    some trees grow brown
     as though saying
       some-
     thing or crying
      maybe and
     only when it's
     too late, nearly
      (if not dead)
     do they question
       "why
  didn't anyone pick up on that?"
       but yet
   the same who ask don't
     see didn't see
  the imminent destruction
    in one they knew—
      so well

SEVENTEEN

One day at my new job my heart arrested when I ran into Julie. The encounter rammed home that whole nightmare I'd been trying to forget. She smiled warmly, recognizing who I was, and when the flail subsided later, I relocated her, my heart in my throat.
   Hi. Are things going any better for you now? *Amazing memory.*
   Oh, not necessarily. I seem to have trouble being who I need to be. But, I just wanted you to have this poem. For whatever . . . *I wanted her to know she'd made the difference—let me feel that maybe one person, at least, didn't detest every inch of me.*

born lovingly
of a green-dense summer morning,
and of my need to share
before it's too late
thank you,
Julie—
for caring those
almost autumn afternoons
when you didn't have to—
for your part
won't ever be forgotten
in antiqued tomorrows
drifting

Any Other Song

> through sun-bright dreams
> of all that we're meant to be and do.
>
> thanks, always—
> for
> caring.

Letting things ride without saying anything was leaving it unfinished, and I had a need to finish things.

Sometime that first, newly different week I had my first appointment with Dr. Bortolli. If I'd had a choice, I would have simply cancelled any further sessions after she meticulously outlined her fees, questioned my income, how often were we supposed to meet, all in a most detached, professional manner.

There'll be a trial period for each of us, of course, as we check each other out to see if we can work together, you know. *And I was expected to entrust myself to her? I'd been spoiled by the warmth and acceptance of Ms Fritz and Greg, and cried all the way back home. The hospital discharge scared me, Dr. Bartolli scared me, work was pressuring. So what if I was supposed to see the woman twice a week! She obviously didn't like me, and came across not even wanting to see me. Like she was really putting herself out to arrange time for me. I keep saying—why don't we all just forget the whole thing? It's not worth it.*

Living alone the first few nights worked out alright, but Dr. Bortolli didn't believe in pills, so each evening after work, I medicated myself with vodka sevens. That way I could rationalize my slow adaptation to singledom, and maybe be so exhausted I wouldn't dream or lie awake agonizing. But the ostracism from Joe and Lindy cut deeper than the depression. I wondered if maybe it hadn't been such a good idea to leave Ted. Granted I had lasted six weeks alone when he was off with Uncle Sam two years before, but I was different then. This time I wasn't making it so well. It didn't even feel as though anyone was there, or even cared. I realized and had to accept that I might not be "the rock," that maybe I never really was, and that I honestly couldn't *do things just because I wanted to badly. Empty promises lost all meaning, always too good to be true. Like being ridiculed for still believing in Santa Claus. Whoever created such magic?*

During my graveyard shift one night, Greg popped in to check on my mental status. I got the crazy notion of trying on him my ambivalence—toying with the idea of moving back in with Ted.

Well. That's your decision, Kathy. I'm sorry to see you're so unsure about the separation, but you've got to take things from where you are now. No more cutting, no more pills. You've got to make a final decision and decide to see it through . . .

It was sort of frightening to hear him being so serious, as though he picked up on the lack of my own understanding for why I'd moved out in the first place. Several days later, hoping for support, I told Jude my intentions.

She was surprised. You know how I feel about Ted. It's like you're throwing away everything we worked to get: an apartment, a car, a new job—and you're tossing it! I'm sorry, Kathy, but this is too much. *And in my tears I lost her.*

Motivated by Jo's piercing pronouncement on my separation, and that Ted felt I'd turned my back on God, as though I were some traitor, I limped back to Ted to seek amends. I approached him the only way I felt was left, trying to be what I thought he wanted. Whatever. However. But one rocky night together wasn't enough to make up for months of bitterness. When I told him a couple of weeks later that I wouldn't be surprised if I was pregnant, he flew apart.

That's just great! Why didn't you warn me?

I just assumed it was alright. I thought that if I did get pregnant, it might help us. At least it would make me feel I could do something positive with myself!

He responded in his typical withdrawn silence. There was really no change—not in him, not between us. It was all the same, just as Jude predicted. I was walking right back into the box that left me no way out. Especially not this time. Maybe not ever. There would be no one to blame but me. I habitually put myself in bad places. But this time, he wasn't especially hot to have me home. So I held off . . .

I forced myself to continue seeing my shrink, hoping it would help, praying it would be enough to keep me going. Trying to burn out the rage and panic, I started jogging. Standing breathless in the middle of a moonlit park, eyes straining up at the stars, I'd yell and scream for God to answer me, to help, to just be there. But all I ever heard was the wind rustling through darkened trees.

On a rainy, foggy Friday afternoon I knew I was losing, and got up enough courage to ask Ms Fritz for help. Because she was right there, right then. I was so taut, babbling on, when I noticed her staring at my umbrella, nearly breaking from my gripping it so fiercely; so I asked for medication, then abruptly realized the absurdity of my entreaty.

Aren't you still seeing your therapist?

Any Other Song

Yeah . . .

Well, I think this is something you should take up with her. When did you last talk to her?

I called her answering service this afternoon, but she still hasn't called me back.

I think you should try again.

But she scares me, and you really seemed to help me!

Kathy, I think that was because you knew there was a time limit on our meetings, and you opened up more than you would have otherwise. *I nodded, slowly, staring at the bare tiled floor, feeling the walls caving in.* Try her again. Ok? I just can't step in.

I knew it wouldn't work, but I had tried. I asked for help this time, and it was refused. Remember that. Just like when I'd gone back to the ward to talk with one of the staff, so I could stabilize myself before going home one night. Those-in-white were too busy, they said. I was no longer their concern. What pathos, because they'd promised that help would always be there when I needed it. All I had to do was ask. Like shit! "Don't you have your own therapist now, Kathy?" *No one was hearing me! Absolutely rejected. And all the people I'd ever loved, listened to, cared about, had drawn the line. C'est tout, madame.*

> *one chandelier summer morning*
> *for just a fleeting moment past*
> *a chinook breeze drifted through the cottonwoods;*
> *for the first time*
> *in an eternity I could see*
> *what togetherness might be with*
> *green-tinged mountains,*
> *the crystalline sky*
> *embroidered with clouds of ivory shawls,*
> *pungent clover fields*
> *scattered with yellow buttercups.*
> *And it was so fine—*
> *as though my nightmares*
> *never were,*
> *as though I was and could be*
> *all that I ever imagined. Jesus,*
> *it was good.*
>
> *but as that essence slipped*
> *out of my tenuous grasp,*
> *I lost everything.*
> *And it*
> *killed me,*
> *because I knew I would never*

E. J. Daniel

*see that soft peace
ever again,
because I'm terrified of the person
I've become and
can't change.*

*and I barely noticed
the gray-black storm explode
over the distant hazy peaks,
the once-warm breeze suddenly chilling.*

*God! what's happened
to me?*

EIGHTEEN

At the ER disguised zoo, Lynne floated in, completely out of control. I couldn't believe she was standing there in the waiting room and hadn't recognized me. I hurried out to help her, to find out what was going on, and ended up escorting her back to the Emergency Psychiatry office and Ms Fritz. She ushered Lynne into one of the consult rooms, and I turned to go back to work, hopeful things were under control, when I saw Lynne bolt out of the room and down the hospital corridor. I started after her, but Ms Fritz stopped me.

Kathy! There's nothing you can do right now. Why don't you just return to work and let us take care of this.

But she's a friend, and she'll listen to me!

We'll take care of it, Kathy. The security guards will pick her up. Please go. *Of course. Call the cops when all else fails.* The line of professionalism had once more been neatly drawn. Ms Fritz had succeeded in making me feel totally incompetent. The anger I'd been denying smashed against my weakening controls as I walked away.

Putting me back together was taking too long, and I grew impatient with the presumption it could even be done at all. Ted wasn't supportive, rattling off endless accusations, planting more barriers to us ever getting differences resolved: "All I want is a sweet,

Any Other Song

thoughtful wife" or "you're just killing yourself by drinking like you do" and "why do you always get us into deeper financial debt?" He did concede a few times to meet me and see Dr. Bortolli. I felt sadly justified that even she appeared frustrated trying to communicate with him. Thankfully he was consistent. She saw through the macho façade he wasn't particularly aware of, then asked me, separately, the big question.

Kathy, with all of your talk of moving back in, have you considered the possibility that Ted might not ever change? Could you live with that?

I didn't know the answer, so I couldn't give any. Could I live with divorce? Could I live, period?

> in the silence
> of a cloudy sky
> on an early evening
> someone lost her
> raison d'être
> and gnashed about
> attempting to rectify
> the grave loss, groping
> for anyone to
> help.
> but in that silence, in
> the loneliness
> there's only
> terror.

The next afternoon, because Greg had said long ago that the games were over, that I was beyond that now, I ripped off some scripts to make my last alternative lethal. I didn't have the courage to jump off a ninth-story balcony like some woman did one Saturday morning during cartoons, nor did I have the means to blow myself to pieces like too many guys I'd known had done. But no more games, remember? I'd even show Brenda that, contrary to her blanket accusation, some people who OD are deadly serious. And the storm continued to escalate, as I waited. I quit caring whether or not I was married—I certainly didn't feel married. Funny. This wasn't how I envisioned things would be years ago... "the jock." Aren't rah-rah's supposed to grow up being everything mothers said they'd be—happily married, making babies, finding gold-potted rainbows? Roles dutifully acted out in high school—protocols—forever lurking around crazy corners. And I'm supposed to be enthralled with the man? Impressed with

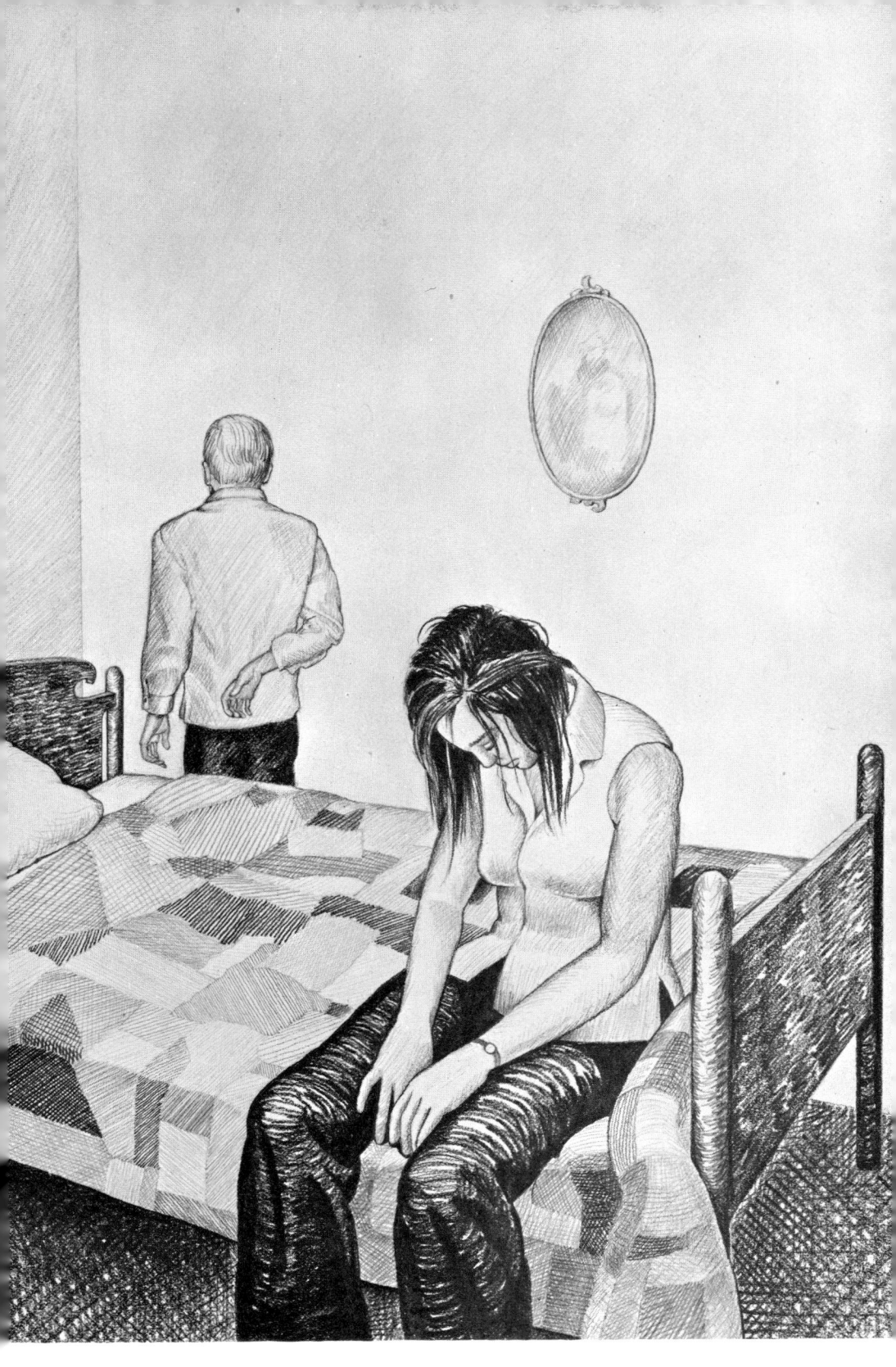

all this? Spare me. But then, I remembered it's not worth the trouble.

When I finally got back to the empty apartment, panic took over. You see, officer, it really happened while she was jogging around the park tonight . . . And the four-in-blue who responded to the hysterical call bustled the lady off to the city hospital to be examined for sexual assault. It wasn't my self who endured the degrading meticulous routine; and when it was over, those-in-white confirmed the alleged rape.

There is a possibility you may already be pregnant. However, we have a couple of alternatives. You can either take the morning-after pill, which will make you sick as a dog for five days, or you can wait and see if you have your period this month. If not, then come on in for an exam when you're a couple of weeks late, and we'll suction you out.

In the middle of the doctor's discourse, Ted appeared in response to those-in-blue's foolish supposition he was needed for moral support. So what if he was already in the house. That little scene axed all of the trust I'd been trying to build back into our damaged relationship. *The dinner I'd arranged to have for him later that week was canceled; we discussed our termination over coffee in the police station cafeteria.*

You know, Kathy. We were never friends. Some strange pathology brought us together, and kept us going for seven rotten years. We never had a healthy interpersonal relationship. You were right saying that I was a "turkey" and a "mouse." I was, but not anymore. I never knew how to say "no" to you, never felt I was strong enough for you. Of course, I'd never have gotten through medical school if you hadn't been pushing me. It'll just be more of the same if we keep seeing each other, so I've decided it'll be less painful for you if we don't. I'm not sure I even like you anymore. There are too many things you've done that I can't ever forgive. *His silence was obviously over.*

Well. Uh, do you want the rings back? Or what?

There you go again! Don't force me into making a decision until I'm ready. I don't agree with divorce, but I've never been closer to getting one. I'll let you know. Oh, by the way, I got my first choice for my internship.

Great. I'm happy for you. One last thing—whether you believe me or not, I'm sorry. God, I'm so sorry it didn't work! *And goodbye. That was it. You threw it all away. Reap what you sow . . .*

I felt compelled to confess to Dr. Bortolli about most of my recent craziness. She was the only one listening; of course, that was her job. I started with the pills.

Any Other Song

I've never run into anything like this before, Kathy. You know that's terribly illegal. *I nodded, staring at my clenched hands, but happy inside I'd finally done something to alarm her. Maybe she'd hear me now.* But, more importantly, I'm worried about your impulsiveness. *Good point. I did tend to be spontaneous.* Do you have the pills with you?

No. *I lied.*

Well, do you think you could find time today to go home and get them, and drop them off in my mailbox?

I studied the tiny room, the worn green carpet, rich paneled walls, the plants in the sunny window silhouetted hazily against the faded blue sky. Why did she have red chairs with green carpet? I ventured to look at her.

Uh, have the police contacted you at all?

What ever do you mean?

I couldn't believe that I was sitting there, telling her about the rape, and about how, when I'd been taken down after the exam to police headquarters at four in the morning, while I'd been giving my report to the mellow Swedish detective, she heard about me having been in too many hospitals. And since I was still in therapy, she would need Dr. Bortolli's verification of my mental instability. I couldn't exactly remember how it all happened, telling different people parts of each story. I didn't want to be there, but the discomfort soon faded as I reminded myself I would soon be dead, so, in a way, the pain didn't matter.

Kathy! You've got to leave your fantasies and games alone if you ever want to stay out of unhealthy and potentially dangerous situations! Are you listening? *She was aghast.*

I guess I'd been rambling, but what she said sounded as though she was admitting I was really psychotic. Inside, I felt a subtle raging growing out of control.

Can I count on you to bring the pills by? *She waited for an answer as I gazed wildly at the floor, my ears ringing. I agreed to bring them by just to get myself out of there, to get her off my back, but I had no intention of giving them to her. That would be admitting it was all a game. And it wasn't. It was for real.*

As I left, I handed her a last-ditch attempt at saying what was going on somewhere inside, because the visiting nurse who follows up on rape victims had encouraged me to try just one more time. For Kathy. What a laugh.

              on any recent dawn
           that i don't care to wake up to

E. J. Daniel

>i sift the meager alternatives
>my mind understands in a
>distant rational way
>but my insides
>scream
>uncontrollably
>"it's a lie!"
>
>you see, doctor,
>i'm afraid of you—
>afraid of what you think and say—
>terrified and tired
>of trying to face another endless
>horror-ridden day.
>i could cry as
>it's just not going to work
>and it never will.
>it makes me sick,
>but i can't
>keep on going,
>anymore . . .

She shook my hand in closure, as usual, saying commandingly, "courage!" and I drifted out of her musty office for the last time, in tears that she'd let me go, just like that. But what else could she do? I couldn't change, I was forever getting into trouble, continually hurting myself and others. People said I could make it in the end, but that wasn't true. Who was I supposed to make it for? Ted would always have his medicine, so where did that leave me?

So I took my little car and the remnants of myself up to the mountains. An afternoon sun was burning away the unwanted sterility of the hospital, intensifying the odor of the sap oozing from the scorched evergreens along the dusty, bumpy road. I let the semi-orange sunset smeared across the sky sear in my mind for an eternity, as everything inside craved to be going with that last malingering warmth. And all I could do was cry, because I finally accepted failure; it would never work. Not for me. Not now. Not ever.

>it's cold outside
>and finally fall
>just like inside
>where answers are lost,
>never found
>and rain
>like tears
>drowns

Any Other Song

>   my mind
>   alone
>   as never before
>   while silent faces watch
>   as i
>   dissolve
>   so it won't hurt—
>   but it does,
>   anyway.

    The next thing I remember, some sheriff was shining his flashlight in my face.
    Hey, lady! You Ok?
    Um, yeah. Just sleepy.
    Well, you can't stay parked here. Maybe you ought to go home.
    I mumbled some reply as I started up the engine, my head leaning against the steering wheel. The sheriff waited for me to move, so, presuming I was already headed in the right direction, I drove off. The moon dreamily illumined the nearby firs and aspen trunks, the intermittent white stripes glowing down the ribboning highway. I vaguely recalled running into and getting plastered with a bunch of motorcycle dudes—what was one more time?—and must have passed out en route home. Or something. I was Ok driving for awhile, barely discerning the semi-familiar landmarks along the winding road, in a timeless dimension, fuzzy treetops washing into a lunar midnight somewhere between alpha and omega.

POSTLUDE

It had been apparent for several weeks that Kathy wasn't coping well. She would come into work slightly intoxicated, pretending to come across as though there was nothing unusual about her behavior. As though no one would notice.

When she first started working there, we were all cautioned to not get involved so we wouldn't feel responsible or guilty if something serious happened to her which we had no control over. Consequently, everyone put a great deal of distance between themselves and Kathy—just to be safe. But Kathy consistently put herself out, waging a subtle war against the staff-imposed isolation, even as she gimped around in a cast. Maybe seeing that side of her was one reason why some of us got involved, anyway. We genuinely wanted to believe in the better, healthy part of her. One morning when Kathy was coming off nights, she admitted how raunchy she felt and what all had happened lately because of her drinking. J. J. was standing in the back with us, and when Kath promised to not ever succumb again, she was hugged out of joyous relief. We really wanted to see her in a better place.

But it didn't last. One chaotic Monday evening Kathy was roaring around work, as usual, when Jourdie drew her aside and asked her if she was on speed. Of course it was denied. But later that night, when J. J. drove into the parking lot before her shift, she spotted Kathy trucking along, going in the opposite direction.

Any Other Song

"Hey, Kath! I was just bringing you a milkshake to help celebrate the end of my class."

"I don't believe it!"

"Where are you going, anyway?"

"Oh, uh—whipping over to get the crew something. It's pretty slow tonight."

"I'll drive you over."

"*No!* That's Ok. I'll just meet you back at work."

"Don't be silly. Get in."

J. J. had wondered why Kathy seemed so hostile; she soon found out why. Kathy hadn't been on her way to get hamburgers, but liquor. She panicked when some doctor who had examined her at City Hospital remembered her while he was doing his rotation with us. Since Kathy subsequently didn't need to be alone that night, J. J. called Jourdie to see if she minded letting Kathy crash there after work. I was unaware of that arrangement when she and I planned to meet each other at a disco later on that evening. J. J. informed me of the plan, though, when I arrived to pick Kathy up and she had already left.

When I finally caught up with Kathy at the bar, she was more out of it than I'd ever seen her. I watched her down a couple of drinks before she told me she had taken even more pills since leaving work. I nearly hurled my glass into the fireplace; I had no idea she had overdosed. I called to warn Jourdie but she refused to let me drive her over there. I should have anyway. She roared out of the parking lot like a screaming banshee; I nearly wrecked my car trying to keep her in sight. By the time I arrived at Jourdie's, Kath was collapsed on the lawn. Jourdie had just found her.

"Kathy! What is going on?"

"I'm sorry. I'm so sorry. I just keep screwing up."

"C'mon. Let's get you inside. How much have you had to drink?"

"Too much . . ."

Jourdie looked at me, deeply concerned. "Kathy, did you take any pills?"

She wouldn't answer. I exploded.

"Damn it, Kath!! How many did you take?"

"Not enough to do anything."

I felt like picking her up and punching her out, I was so angry.

"Kathy. We're going to have to take you in to the Emergency Room and pump you out." Jourdie was nearly crying. "You haven't left us any other choice. I can't be sure you haven't really taken too many, especially with all the alcohol you've had."

Tears streamed down Kathy's face as she begged us not to take

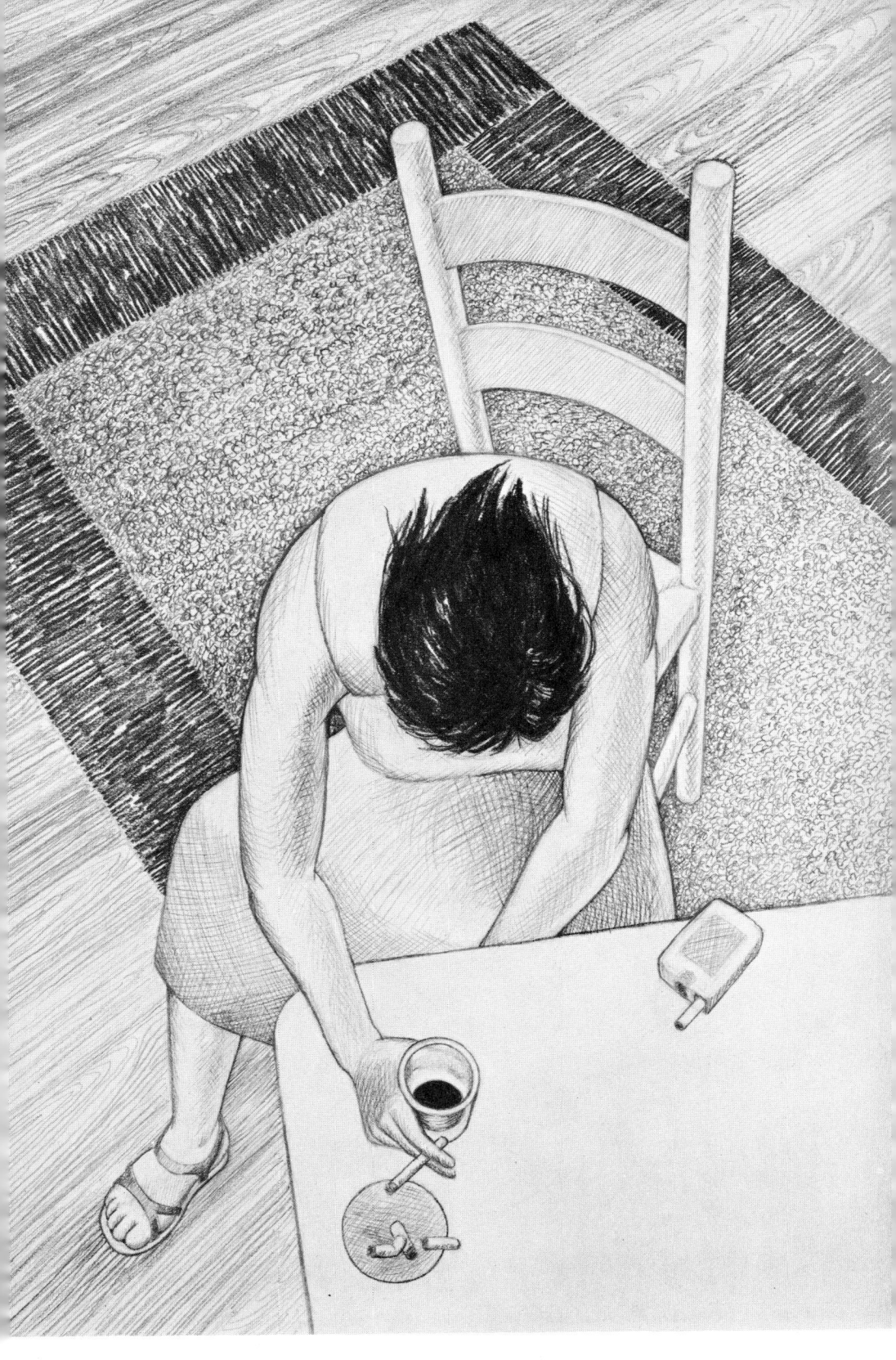

her, swearing she'd only swallowed five more of the 30mg Dalmane we'd found her popping in the bathroom and "maybe a few aspirin to ward off a headache." It was well past 1 AM as we walked her into the kitchen to fill her full of coffee and grape juice. When it was impossible to keep her awake any longer, we put her in bed, not at all convinced we'd done the best thing. I stayed over, and unable to sleep, strained to hear the sound of her depressed breathing as I lay beside her.

Morning couldn't come soon enough. Kathy remained withdrawn and silently hung over as we drove her to see her psychiatrist. It was an uncomfortable session for all of us, Kathy sobbingly apologizing at Dr. Bortolli's insistence, reiterating how sorry she was for having done that to us.

"Kathy, I hope you now realize that this isn't what friends are for. It puts an awful strain on the relationship. You're terribly fortunate to have such people care about you so greatly . . ."

> words adequate
> or not
> to say where i'm at
> or not
> sadly thanking anyone
> not enough
> for well-intended concern that
> can't stop
> the part of me
> hell-bent on
> destruction
> having tried no less than
> seven times before but
> too many
> failures
> or was that God
> intervening
> for whatever purpose?
>
> and i'm scared,
> i think,
> for who'll win
> this
> time?

The most difficult action the three of us have ever been faced with was prompted by Kathy's behavior over the next couple of days. She'd assured us things were better and more in control, but after we heard about her Wednesday follow-up appointment with her doc and how

Any Other Song

she'd spent the following 24 hours roaring through the mountains, Jourdie made arrangements to spend the night with her on Thursday. Before J. J. left work, I decided to stop by and share some leftover pizza with them; it was Kathy's favorite. But I ended up hanging around until Jourdie got there to take Kath home. Luckily there was sufficient staffing so that she wasn't really needed. Not that Kathy was even functioning. When she finally realized I was there, she stumbled over and hugged me hello for nearly five minutes, standing immobile in the back hallway, oblivious to the pizza—or anything else. Her affect was totally inappropriate, and in response to her vibes, I pocketed some ipecac to give Jourdie as we piled Kathy into the car.

My out-of-town friend was not exactly understanding of the situation, especially when, the following morning, I decided I needed to check on Kathy before he and I were to head into the mountains. I ran into J. J. on the way up the front steps, both of us becoming grim when Jourdie met us at the door, exhausted and crying.

"What's happened?"

"Oh, you guys! I've been up all night with her. She must've taken at least 30 or 40 Dalmane, the aspirin bottle's empty, on top of who knows how much booze. After the ipecac, I didn't get her to bed until five this morning, and then couldn't sleep I was so afraid she'd arrest."

I was furious. "Where is she?"

"Fixing breakfast, as though nothing's happened. I don't see how."

"So what are we going to do?"

"The only thing left." We looked at each other, hating to make such a decision, but caring too much not to. The hardest part was knowing that action was the one thing Kathy vowed would never happen to her again. But we had no other choice . . .

A wasted Jourdie had to work days, and as she got ready, I tried to contact Dr. Bortolli; J. J., attempting a conversation with Kathy, swept out of the kitchen in tears.

"She's not even aware of what's going on. It's crazy!"

Breakfast was a joke. I told Kathy we had called her doc, who agreed with our decision for hospitalization. She looked at us incredulously before slamming into the bedroom. I charged after her as Jourdie made a late exit.

"Pack, Kathy!"

"There's no way I'm going! No way!"

"Like hell! Now get your things together and let's get going."

"Why can't I just spend the day with J. J. like we'd planned? It'll be alright."

"Not a chance. And I'll fight you if I have to! Now, pack." I couldn't believe the utter contempt and hostility in her eyes.

As we walked Kathy to the hospital, a group of nurses heading in the opposite direction passed by. One of them greeted Kath, but she wouldn't respond. Sighing, I shook my head. J. J. continued her contemplation of the sidewalk.

Just inside the building, Kathy abruptly stopped; she was fighting to the bitter end.

"What are you doing?" J. J. was fighting back.

"I don't have to do this!"

"Damn it, Kathy! Don't you see how much it's hurting us? Now, come on!" I had never seen J. J. cry, but she was past her limit. We all were.

Kath stared at the floor as she stalked past us and sat down in the conference room. While we silently awaited her shrink, the nurse we passed on the way poked her head in.

"Karin!" Her entrance was immediately palliative.

"Hi, Kathy. I thought you might be here. The look you gave me bothered me so much I had to excuse myself from the discussion and come find you." With that, Kath fell apart, and I left, it hurt so much.

Outside, I asked one of the psych nurses what would happen next. At least Dr. Bortolli had called to authorize Kathy's hospitalization. I followed the staff nurse back into the small conference room, and stood in the corner as she read the 72-hour hold to Kathy. Not surprisingly, she refused to sign.

> IN THE PROBATE COURT, IN AND FOR THE STATE, IN THE INTEREST OF
> Kathleen Brooke, I, Leslie Weston, RN, MS, a peace officer, licensed physician, certified psychologist or other mental health professional affirm that, as a result of personal observations or as a result of information obtained from others which I believe to be reliable, have probable cause to believe that the above Respondent:
> 1) appears to be mentally ill *AND*
> 2) an imminent danger to herself.
>
> The conditions and facts which indicate that the patient should be held for 72 hour treatment and evaluation are: that she took 20 sleeping pills and an unknown amount of ETOH last night in an attempt to kill herself. She did this when she was with friends but did not inform them. This a.m. she refuses hospitalization, states she would be 'with a friend.' No circumstances have changed. Her treating physician agrees an involuntary hold is necessary because of continued suicidal risk.

By mid-afternoon we said our goodbyes to Kathy as she stood stiffly inside the door of the psych ward.

Any Other Song

"We're really sorry, Kath, but there just wasn't anything else we could do . . ." It felt even worse as she shrugged in defeat and turned away without even looking at us. We went down to the cafeteria to meet Jourdie for her break. No one said anything as we stared into our coffee, wishing that day had never happened.

> Admit Note: Kathy is a 25-year-old white female, wife of a senior medical student, who was referred to me in May from this hospital for outpatient treatment after a hospitalization for an OD. Her ideation, plans, verbalization, have intermittently been centered on self-defeating behavior and suicide. Thursday night she took 40 Dalmane (30 mg), an unknown amount ASA and ETOH, after stating in my office earlier in the week that nothing anyone could do would help and that she just had "some loose ends to tie up." We contracted that she would call me regarding her decision about the meds she told me she had *(I have not prescribed anything at all for her)*. I checked back with her last night since she had not called, but no answer. I would like the team to give primary care (since, if there is a way, Kathy will manage to fall between two chairs) but I will remain available for consultation and follow-up after discharge.

> *yuccas and windmills*
> *etch endless horizons*
> *—no screaming here,*
> *please! Sunsets*
> *smear forever skies of*
> *foggy dawn to faded dusk*
> *yet—*
> *love reaches*
> *inside*
> *as your sacrificial rainbow*
> *softly warms*
> *my sometime*
> *self. . .*

But, you know, Kath, some of us—we hear, we hurt—not because you have the power to inflict pain on us, but we cry because we choose to. If only you could let yourself hear that . . .

> *on the other side of summer*
> *grass green*
> *before the sun*
> *created parchment and*
> *dreams fantastic then*
> *grew sadly sobered*

E. J. Daniel

*but
because time's sifting so long
salt still runs
down those lonely
stale summer
afternoons.*

CONSIDER

1. Who is ultimately responsible to care for a person whose illness becomes bothersome or embarrassing to those involved (i.e., patient, health professional, or others)?
2. Davis* writes that "the question of suicide is extremely controversial in our society and raises many ethical questions for the health professional about the individual's right to self-determination versus the right of the human community to preserve itself. Whose rights should prevail in the face of conflict?" Her question also raises the question of protocol—on what basis would the health professional decide to intervene, and at what level?
3. How objective can the health professional be in treating patients with whom they are subjectively involved?

---

*Davis, A and Aroskar, M. Ethical Dilemmas and Nursing Practice. *New York: Appleton-Century-Crofts, 1978, p. 125.*